# CESAREAN CHILDBIRTH

## A Handbook For Parents

*CHRISTINE COLEMAN WILSON
AND
WENDY ROE HOVEY*

DOLPHIN BOOKS
Doubleday & Company, Inc., Garden City, New York   1980

To Our Families

| Rob | Joe |
|---|---|
| Jonathan | Brian |
| Adrienne | Rebecca |

All illustrations by Lewis L. Sadler

Library of Congress Cataloging in Publication Data

Wilson, Christine Coleman.
  Cesarean childbirth.

  Bibliography: p. 283
  Includes index.
  1. Cesarean section.   I. Hovey, Wendy Roe, joint
author.   II. Title. [DNLM: 1. Cesarean section—
Handbooks. WQ430 W747c]
RG761.W49      618.8′6
ISBN: 0-385-15154-3
Library of Congress Catalog Card Number 78–22792

# ACKNOWLEDGMENTS

Writing a book is much harder than we imagined. And the support and criticism of others are not merely helpful, they are also essential if the book is to be more than just a personal diatribe. Although we take full responsibility for the contents of this book, we want to thank the following people who helped us as we worked.

Rob and Joe—we knew that you believed in us and that you wanted this to be a good book. What we didn't know until it was too late is that you would have to survive large doses of single parenthood, that this project was basically insane, that two women with four small children between them should never undertake to write a book. Thank you for the kinds of support that none of us knew would be needed, but that in the end made it all possible.

George Nolan, in the five years of our association we have been strengthened by your belief in us and enriched by the kind of person and physician you are. You never doubted the importance of what we were trying to do, even though we had so many doubts. You have always understood what we know now, that parents and children are the main actors in the childbearing drama, while the professionals are the supporting cast. Thank you for the innumerable ways in which you have supported us.

Many people have shared their own personal experiences with us, and those are the greatest gifts they could have given. We remain forever indebted to the group of women whose concerns were the foundation for the original booklet, which in turn led us to write this book. We are grateful to the many parents and professionals who wrote to us after the original booklet was published to share their experiences and their viewpoints. Special thanks go to David and Marie Rees, Betsy and Pat Risen, and Pat and Jim Vernon, who gave something of themselves to us.

Many people shared their knowledge about a particular area, or critically read some portion of the manuscript and commented on it. For this we thank Sarah H. Broman, Ph.D; Valmai Howe Elkins, R.P.T.; Avis J. Ericson, Pharm.D.; Edward Grandt, M.D.; Greg Henry, M.D.; Jon Homuth, M.D.; Karen Micas, M.S.W.; Cornelia DeSocio, R.N., B.S.Ed., P.N.P.; David Webb, M.D.; Gregory White, M.D.; and Mary White.

Other friends and associates contributed their time and talents in important ways. We are thankful to the staff of Arnot-Ogden Memorial Hospital, Elmira, New York, and especially to Sue Dana, Katherine Mekos, and medical photographer Mike Sheehe. Lois Maschmeyer read and critiqued the entire manuscript. Barbara Softcheck and Susan Stelter gave support and encouragement. Eleanor Funk was always available to hear our concerns. And last but not least, our editor, Karen Van Westering, guided us through the maze of the publishing world and saw to it that we emerged relatively unscathed.

# CONTENTS

# PREFACE

When Chris was told that she had to have a Cesarean delivery, it came as a great shock. Her first baby had been an easy vaginal delivery. A year later, when Wendy had her first child by Cesarean, the stage was set. We didn't know each other yet, but the beginnings of our friendship and this book lay in those two birth experiences.

Chris took the first step with a brief blurb in a local newsletter. It simply said that she had some feelings about her Cesarean birth experience, and wondered if anyone else did, and if so, did anyone want to talk about it? Wendy jumped at the chance, and we set a time to meet. Two of the other women who responded couldn't come to the meeting at the last minute. The third just never showed up. So the two of us shared our birth experiences, and wondered if we were a little strange for feeling the way we did then.

But Chris's phone kept ringing, and it soon became obvious that there were lots of women who had had Cesareans and wanted to tell someone about it who also had been through it. Others were feeling tired, disappointed, and depressed, and they were looking for support. Some just appreciated the chance to socialize and show off their babies. Many wanted more information about what had happened to them. And, from the start, women called to say, "How can I make it better the next time?"

We worked together gathering information on Cesarean birth. We talked to doctors, childbirth educators, and hospital administrators. We spent time in libraries and viewed films. The more we found out, the more questions we had. We depended heavily on medical experts, yet there were many times when the experts did not agree. And we found that we had a kind of expertise the experts did not: We had experienced Cesarean childbirth.

We decided that the wealth of information we had compiled would be helpful to other couples who had a Cesarean birth. Our first booklet *Cesarean Childbirth: A Handbook for Parents* slowly took shape. ("Slowly" is the important word—the project took us a couple of years.) We balanced family demands and authorship, and found that dining-room tables are not inspiring work areas, particularly when they must be cleared to make room for the hungry hordes three times a day. Wendy moved to New York State, and the phone bills began to climb. But we finished it at last, and had it printed ourselves. Then came the slow process of distributing the booklet from our homes.

Gradually, word spread and our booklet sales increased steadily. Because the original booklet was so successful, we were encouraged to accept the opportunity to write this book. In fact, we were dazzled by the opportunity to say everything that we didn't have enough space for in the original booklet, and to get out of the promotion and distribution business!

So in late 1978 we began again, this time *knowing* that these words would eventually see a printing press. It was even more complicated this time. Wendy had just had a second Cesarean baby and was busy with a private practice in counseling. Chris's children had reached "middle age" and she had begun teaching and taking courses in preschool education. But we wrote, and talked by phone (Ma Bell loves us), and spent many weekends together lovingly tearing apart each other's prose. As we worked, we became painfully aware of the politics of childbearing, the complexity of the issues, and the variety of Cesarean birth experiences. Uppermost in our minds was a desire to write a book for all Cesarean parents that would be helpful whether they were preparing for their child's birth or viewing it in retrospect.

Over the past years, we have become increasingly aware of the role that informed and responsible consumers can play in all phases of medical care. We experienced this process firsthand when we became involved in the discussions with our local hospital that eventually led to fathers being permitted to attend Cesarean births. Inevitably, our experiences as consumers merged with our perspectives as parents.

This book is from two women who have experienced Cesarean birth to all Cesarean parents and parents-to-be. We believe that information is the key to acceptance and to change. With this book, we celebrate your curiosity, your concern, and your commitment to joyful Cesarean birth.

November 1979

# INTRODUCTION

Cesarean section, a surgical method of childbirth, is today a topic of much discussion and concern. Many of the reasons why Cesareans were controversial in the past have been resolved, making this method of birth very safe. These factors (better surgical techniques, antibiotics, blood transfusions, etc.), which have made the operation safe, have also contributed to an increased number of births by this route. Many couples who embark upon childbearing today are aware of challenges, by professionals, consumers, and governmental groups, to all aspects of Cesarean birth. The couples often feel anxiety because of the uncertainty over these unresolved issues. Resolution of these issues may take many years, but couples starting families now cannot wait.

The authors in writing this book have sought to fill a gap between medicine and consumer. They have recognized that a Cesarean birth represents a crisis, and while they have been unable to change that fact, they have identified and discussed many aspects of surgical births that intensify the crisis for most parents. Learning about and understanding what is involved when a Cesarean birth occurs can be of enormous value to parents. This book provides that information, and its contents reflect the enormous understanding and effort put forth by Ms. Hovey and Ms. Wilson. They have addressed the important issues in a straightforward manner and have shown significant objectivity in areas that are controversial. They have been careful to distinguish opinion from fact.

The authors have written in a style that allows the reader to relax while getting a thorough exposure to the important facts and issues about Cesarean birth. The book's contents range from trends in obstetrics to parent-infant bonding. In the slang of today, they "tell it like it is." But unlike many writers today in dealing with issues, they place things in perspective. The book addresses and answers most of the questions couples ask physicians and nurses, and it answers many that patients are afraid or reluctant to ask. It bridges the gap between what physicians routinely say and what patients want and need to know. It is written in an accessible style by two women who are knowledgeable about the subject and who have experienced Cesarean births themselves. It is written by women who feel and care.

I recommend this book to physicians, nurses, and students of the subject, but most of all, to those for whom it was intended: couples bearing children.

GEORGE H. NOLAN, M.D.
Associate Professor, Obstetrics and Gynecology
University of Michigan Medical Center
Ann Arbor, Michigan

# ONE

# Childbirth Today— Issues and Trends

You probably remember the moment when you first learned you were pregnant. The voice on the telephone said, "The test results were positive." Hooray! But now what?

Your preparation for parenthood takes many forms. There are clothes and equipment to be bought, decisions to be made, and feelings about yourself to be absorbed.

> My mind was in a whirl. I wanted to leave work and run over to Jack's office to tell him, so I could see his face. I started planning for how to get the room ready, imagining different ways to arrange the furniture. But thinking about the furniture brought me face to face with the fact that my income was going to stop in eight months. How would we pay for all of this? Then I started trying to picture the baby, imagining first a boy and then a girl. I decided I really didn't care which one it was. Just let it be OK; that's all that matters.

In addition, most couples now have some formal preparation for the actual birth. Doctors often recommend childbirth classes, and they are usually required if the couple wishes to be together when the baby is born.

My neighbor wanted to know if I was going to "go natural" when I had the baby. I said I was, but I was thinking to myself that I really didn't know what it meant to "go natural." I wondered if I could do it and if it hurt a lot. I started to ask my neighbor, but then I remembered that she had both of hers by Cesarean.

The experience of childbirth has changed radically since the turn of the century. Your grandmother may have allowed herself to wonder if she would live through the birth of each succeeding child. Your mother didn't need to worry so much about survival, but she probably hoped for enough medication from the doctor to be spared the agonies of childbirth. But couples who have children now dream of a birth experience that is not only safe and relatively free of pain, but also emotionally rewarding. They see the birth of the baby as a culmination of all their dreams throughout the nine months of pregnancy. They wish to share the birth, though each may have his or her private fears about how this partnership will withstand the event. They want to feel as much in charge and in control as they can. And they expect to be rewarded for all their practice and preparation at the moment when the baby is born, and they can greet her, touch her, and make her their own.

However, at the same time that childbirth preparation has come into its own, another obstetrical revolution has been under way. The rate of Cesarean births in the United States tripled in the ten years from 1965 to 1975. Unfortunately, most couples prepare for only one form of birth. When they have an unexpected Cesarean instead, their pain and fear are at least as great as for women decades ago. In fact, they may be much greater, because the couples approached the birth with such high hopes.

People kept coming in and listening and looking and retreating to the hall and muttering. My doctor came in and said that I would have a Cesarean. I didn't know what in the hell that meant. Someone brought me papers to sign. Someone took blood samples. Someone attached an IV. Someone attached a catheter. I lost sight of my husband in the mass of people around me. I lost sight of the fact I was having a baby. I was just a prone body with wires running from a lot of directions.

Until very recently, childbirth preparation and Cesarean birth were on a collision course. To many couples, and to childbirth educators and health care professionals as well, the two seemed mutually exclusive. Now we are beginning to understand that there can be prepared Cesarean birth that can bring the same rewards as a planned vaginal delivery.

The rapid increase in the Cesarean birthrate is highly controversial. In an area where the experts disagree, what can the consumer do? This is a book for parents, and some of the answers to "What can you do?" depend on the stage of parenthood you are in now. If you are pregnant, you can make sure that your childbirth preparation includes complete knowledge about both vaginal and Cesarean birth, and also about your rights and responsibilities as a medical consumer. If you have already had a Cesarean, you can educate yourself in order to understand what happened to you and deal with your feelings about the experience. Perhaps you are beginning to plan for your next birth, at the same time. Even if you have decided that your family is complete, you still may be one of the many Cesarean couples who feels a strong need to understand their birth experience.

I kept thinking of more things to ask the doctor. But my six-week checkup was done and I didn't want to bother him on the phone. Before I could decide what to do, I ran across a book that showed pictures of a Cesarean. Right after that, there was a TV show about it. The show was about whether there are too many sections, but the part I cared about was seeing it happen. It showed the whole thing and I wasn't even bothered. In a way, I think it gave me some peace about it.

## THE RISING CESAREAN RATE

In 1965, the rate of Cesarean births was about 4.5 per cent of all births. By 1975, it had increased to 12 to 15 per cent for most hospitals and 20 to 25 per cent in many large medical centers.

(Some facilities report rates much higher than these.) During each of the past three years approximately 400,000 babies were born by Cesarean delivery.

Why are so many more Cesareans being done? Some reasons are easy to identify. Some are more complex. Many are causing controversy among medical professionals and parents alike. Part of the explanation lies in the fact that Cesarean deliveries are much safer now than they were a decade ago. Improvements in the operation itself and in anesthesia techniques, along with the development of blood banks and antibiotics, have significantly reduced many of the risks that were once feared when a Cesarean delivery was necessary. While surgical birth is still riskier than vaginal delivery—because it is indeed a major operation—it is now a very safe way to have a baby.

The rise in Cesarean births can be partially explained too by the greater emphasis on the well-being of every baby who is delivered. Many couples are choosing to limit the number of children they have. Each child is a very special individual. Parents and doctors wish to make every effort to insure that the baby has a full, healthy life. As they work toward this goal, many may feel that a Cesarean delivery is preferable to a vaginal delivery that would involve even the smallest risk to the baby. This philosophy marks a major change in attitude toward Cesarean birth. Formerly surgical deliveries were done only to correct an existing problem—for example, a baby that was just too large to pass through the vaginal canal. Now a Cesarean is often done so that a potential problem can be avoided.

The current practice of delivering almost all breech (feet or buttocks first) babies by Cesarean is an example of this change in attitude. Some studies have shown a much higher percentage of problems in breech babies who were delivered vaginally than in those who were in the vertex (head first) position. Yet it is still true that most breech babies who were delivered vaginally are perfectly healthy. Since there is no way at present to know which breech babies might have problems, many doctors would prefer to deliver all by Cesarean and avoid such risks.

There are other changes in medical practice that have added to the increase in Cesarean births. Many doctors now feel that unless a woman will have a relatively easy and fast vaginal birth, a Cesarean delivery is probably preferable. For instance, some doctors believe that the risks involved in surgical delivery are much lower than those present if forceps are needed to help deliver a baby. Yet there is legitimate disagreement about what constitutes a difficult vaginal delivery—difficult enough to be worth avoiding in favor of the risks of surgery.

It is also often necessary to deliver the babies of women with certain medical conditions (such as diabetes or hypertension) before full term. With sophisticated neonatal care now available, these babies may be better off in the intensive care nursery than they would be in the uterus, even when they are delivered prematurely. Since it is often very difficult to induce successful labor before your due date, Cesarean delivery is necessary.

As more women have Cesarean deliveries with their first babies, repeat Cesarean procedures continue to increase accordingly. Most obstetricians feel that one Cesarean birth means that all subsequent children must be surgically delivered. Although more doctors are beginning to allow a trial of labor for selected women, this is still a highly controversial matter. Until more women are allowed to try a vaginal delivery after Cesarean birth, the sheer numbers of women who have repeat Cesareans will continue to escalate.

Unfortunately, there are times when a Cesarean is done to protect the doctor as well as the mother and the baby. Suits have been filed and judgments won by parents who said a Cesarean should have been done when it wasn't. It is impossible to say how many "defensive" Cesareans are currently being done. It is certainly a matter of concern to parents and doctors alike.

In the face of the skyrocketing use of surgery to deliver babies, responsible professionals and consumers are asking how many of these Cesareans are really necessary. When each Cesarean is evaluated individually, virtually all seem justified. With very few exceptions, a doctor who was assessing the work of another would find that, although he or she might not have made the same decision under the same circumstances, he or she can see the validity of each decision that was made. Yet taken as a nationwide trend, the Cesarean rate seems very high—too high in many people's view. The word "iatrogenic" means "an error induced by medical or surgical treatment." We may assume that some Cesareans are iatrogenic. But how many and which ones?

Some critics of the high Cesarean rate have accused the growing practice of routine electronic fetal monitoring of being the iatrogenic villain. It is true that the rise in Cesarean births corresponds with the introduction of monitors. Yet so many other changes were going on in obstetrics at the same time that it would be impossible to identify which trends were caused by others.

A similar concern arises around the practice of rupturing women's membranes in order to hasten labor. Some critics fear that obstetricians have become so overconcerned with the desirability of labor being "progressive" that they may rupture the membranes before nature is ready to begin labor in earnest. Since most doctors feel that a delivery by some route must occur within twenty-four hours from the time the membranes are ruptured, a Cesarean may result.

## FACING THE DILEMMA

What is an acceptable Cesarean rate? Not long ago, one measure of high-quality maternity care was a Cesarean rate of not more than 5 per cent. Doctors who did Cesareans more frequently than one birth out of twenty were subject to the scrutiny of their peers. Now, the norm has risen to around 12 to 15 per cent. Instead of one out of twenty, one out of seven babies are born surgically. In the face of such rapidly changing standards of practice, how does the pregnant couple protect themselves from being caught at the far side of the pendulum's swing?

Complete preparation for both kinds of birth is part of the answer. The reason that the prepared childbirth movement has become so widespread is that it offers tangible benefits to consumer and professional alike. For the consumer, the benefits are knowledge, training, and confidence.

> Before we took the classes, I couldn't imagine what it would be like to have the baby. I remember asking my friend Gloria to describe a contraction for me, and I just couldn't connect with the answer she gave me. Now we have been to five classes. I still don't really know what a contraction is going to be like, but I feel different about it. I guess the difference is, no matter what a contraction is, I know what to do about it when I start feeling one for the first time.

For many parents, the most important advantage to taking childbirth preparation classes is that the classes restore their sense of autonomy. These couples place a strong value on being in charge of their own destiny. The classes give them the tools they need to feel in charge, even though they are facing something totally new and somewhat unpredictable.

Many childbirth educators now tell each new group of pregnant couples, "At least one of you will have a Cesarean birth." Each couple nods uncomfortably and silently hopes it will be someone else. This is understandable; almost no one would choose surgery if it could be avoided. But there is more than the fear of surgery for many couples. It is their fear that they will lose all the benefits of childbirth preparation if they must have a Cesarean. They want to feel knowledgeable, trained, and prepared, and they believe that they cannot approach Cesarean birth in that way. There is even a bit of illogic at work here: "If we don't think about it, then it won't happen." Unfortunately, it is often the very couples who ignore the possibility of a Cesarean birth who have the most difficult time adjusting if it becomes a reality.

> My husband and I had really prepared for this birth. We read every book about childbirth we could get our hands on. We had gone to classes and movies, on hospital tours, and talked with friends. We had practiced breathing patterns until we felt we could do them in our sleep. When our doctor told us a Cesarean would be necessary, we just couldn't understand. That was not part of anything we had

learned or come to expect from this childbirthing business we had entered. We needed someone to tell us why everything we had hoped for was falling apart.

## WOMEN'S CHANGING VIEWS ABOUT THEMSELVES

For years, many women related to their doctors in a dependent way, asking the doctor to take charge and make many decisions for them. In fact, some of the medical practices that women now find most objectionable gained their original acceptance twenty or thirty years ago, when women counted on their doctors to make childbirth as painless as possible. "Twilight sleep" and induced labors were greeted as wonderful aids for the then-modern mother-to-be.

As women work toward a greater degree of self-determination, health care—especially where reproduction and childbearing are concerned—has become a major issue. Most women use some form of birth control, making childbirth a matter of choice, not destiny. In addition, knowledge about good nutrition and prenatal care is becoming widespread. As women take more responsibility for themselves, they also look for ways to increase their control over their reproductive experience.

I remember that my mother always got yelled at by the doctor when she was pregnant for gaining too much weight. She would just take it—and then go eat anyway. When my doctor suggested that I diet, I decided to take him on about it. I showed him some things I had read that said pregnant women should not be on a diet. We talked it over, and I explained that I was very careful not to eat junk. He and I finally agreed that he would not bug me or lecture me unless he felt there really was some danger, and I agreed again to be sensible and not stuff myself.

If a woman is not knowledgeable about Cesarean birth, then she may worry that having a Cesarean will completely undermine her newfound sense of independence. This contributes to some women pretending it can't happen to them. On the other hand, she may recognize the value of preparing for a Cesarean, but meet opposition from her doctor. Even those obstetricians who most welcomed the changes in women's attitudes toward them may feel reluctant to discuss highly technical and possibly frightening issues with their patients.

> We were going along pretty well. Then about the third appointment I asked him what he thought about monitors. He frowned and asked me why I wanted to know. I thought it was just a simple question. All I wanted to know was whether the hospital uses the monitors on everyone right away. When he started answering, I realized how little I knew. He said they use them for everyone who is induced. So then I wanted to know why someone would be induced. That was a whole long discussion in itself. The next time I came in he said, "Here's the lady with all the questions." I couldn't tell from the way he said it whether he thought it was good or not.

Given a choice, many women do not want to be protected from information that may be unpleasant for them to hear. They know that they have the strength to cope with whatever they must. In fact, they have learned that being prepared for every possibility gives them even greater strength.

## THE PREGNANT COUPLE AS MEDICAL CONSUMERS

When couples meet with their doctor there is often an unspoken dialogue taking place. The couple is saying: We need to trust you since you have the expertise we do not possess. We want a healthy baby more than anything in the whole world and we would prefer to have the most natural pregnancy and birth possible. We are afraid something will happen to interfere with our dreams. We are afraid that you might push us into things that we really do not want to do. We are frightened at giving you so much control over something that is so central to our lives.

Doctors are saying: I want you to have confidence in me without thinking that I am omniscient and totally infallible. I want you to believe that I will help you through this pregnancy, giving you the best care possible based on my education, experience, and concern for your health as well as that of your baby. I want you to understand what I am doing and why I am doing it but I don't want you to tell me that you will not accept my advice when I feel in my best judgment it is necessary. I want to co-operate with you as we plan this birth, but I don't know if I can place my trust in you. We seem to have the beginning of a good relationship, but how will you react if something does not work out as all of us would wish?

All of these things—your fears, your dreams, your ability to cope with the health care system—have to be juggled as you work toward truly prepared childbirth.

As you go through pregnancy, you are adding many new roles to your repertoire. Sometimes couples focus on preparing to be parents, without giving enough attention to their new role as medical consumers. If you have only had routine health care until now, then you have a lot to learn about yourself and about the organization and delivery of obstetrical care in North America.

I saw an article in our paper about a birth room that had just been started in our local hospital. It explained that it was opened in response to requests from the community for a more "natural" setting in which to deliver a baby. I guess I had never really thought much about what would happen when we actually got to the hospital before reading that.

Your first responsibility as a consumer is to become knowledgeable. Gather as much information as you can about pregnancy and birth, including all aspects of Cesarean birth. You may find that the more you learn, the more questions you have. In addition to the general kinds of information available in bookstores, there are specific practices that are typical in your area that you will want to become familiar with. And if this is not your first pregnancy, you will find that there have been some changes just since your last child was born.

The town where Nathan and Adam were born was so small. There was just the one hospital and one group of doctors. The care was very personal, but so conservative. We moved before Laura's birth to a pretty big city. I liked my new doctor a lot, but he sure handled things differently. This time I had ultrasound and some other tests. And when I told him that my old doctor said no sex and no salt after the seventh month, he laughed!

Your next responsibility is to discuss your questions thoroughly with your doctor. Valmai Elkins, in her excellent book *The Rights of the Pregnant Parent,* suggests that you open discussions of medical questions with your doctor by asking, "What do you think of . . . ?" This encourages your doctor to share his or her expertise with you, and is likely to result in a much more useful discussion than if you walk into the office with a list of demands. You and your doctor may not always agree, but discussing issues that are currently controversial will give you a chance to become familiar with your doctor's opinions and usual practices. At the same time, it will help your doctor to be sensitive to areas that are of concern to you.

Your final responsibility as a consumer is to make sure that you obtain and participate fully in the best available medical care. It may be difficult to evaluate your doctor's performance on some levels. Medical care often involves highly technical decisions that can require great time and effort on your part if you are to understand what is happening. You can certainly make some judgment about whether your doctor is individualizing your care, partly based on your feeling that he or she is talking to you as an individual rather than that you are the fourth appointment. The best obstetricians are very concerned about the question of what is sound treatment and what is medical interference. When neither the doctor nor the patient insists on rigid answers, then you have the foundation for a professional/consumer partnership.

We all want healthy babies. We all would like to have a healthy birth experience too. Cesarean birth can give us both.

## TWO

# Why a Cesarean Delivery?

Why was our baby born by Cesarean? This question occurs to almost all couples who have experienced surgical delivery. At times the answer is very clear. In most instances, however, the answer is not that absolute. The cause of any particular Cesarean is probably a combination of factors, none of which by themselves would have made the Cesarean necessary. If, for instance, your baby was a bit large and showed some signs of fetal distress and if your pelvis was a bit small, you may have had a Cesarean delivery.

The first Cesarean comes as a total surprise to most couples. It is usually very difficult at the time a Cesarean is announced for your doctor to thoroughly explain what is happening, although some explanation is certainly due you. If the Cesarean is a true emergency, you may find that everyone seems to be rushing off in a thousand different directions, leaving you alone with your concerns. When a Cesarean becomes necessary after a long labor, you may be very tired and unable to comprehend exactly what your doctor is telling you. Often, too, what is being said is that a vaginal delivery might be possible, but in your doctor's best judgment, a Cesarean delivery would be safest for your baby and possibly for you.

This chapter discusses the most common reasons (you may hear them referred to as indications) for Cesarean delivery. A few are absolute, and if any of these conditions appear in your pregnancy, it is almost certain you will have a Cesarean. Many are not that well defined. Obstetrics is an art as well as a science, and our discussion will point out ways in which different doctors might use the same data to come to different conclusions.

## PRIOR CESAREAN DELIVERY

More Cesarean deliveries occur because of previous delivery by Cesarean than for any other reason. A recent study of 120,684 Cesarean deliveries found that 30 per cent were due to "delivery complicated by previous Cesarean section."[1] As more women have Cesarean deliveries with their first child, a proportionately larger number of repeat Cesareans are being done. If the primary (first time) Cesarean rate levels off or drops, the number of repeat surgical deliveries would be lowered also.

Since early in this century, the general rule in the United States has been that once a woman had a Cesarean delivery all subsequent children would be delivered surgically. The "once a Cesarean, always a Cesarean" rule is subject to increasing debate. Studies are under way to evaluate vaginal delivery after Cesarean birth. Women whose first Cesarean was due to a problem unlikely to recur in future pregnancies are asking their doctors for a trial of labor.

When I found out that I was pregnant again I just accepted the fact that I would have another Cesarean delivery. Then I read about

[1] J. A. Lowe, and D. F. Klassen, "Time Trends in U. S. PAS Hospitals in Cesarean Section Rates," *PAS Reporter*, Special Issue, Vol. 14 (Dec. 1976). This report is an extremely thorough assessment of what is happening with Cesarean deliveries in United States hospitals. It includes information on why Cesareans are being done, what type of anesthesia is employed, complications resulting from the procedures, and other pertinent data.

some women who had vaginal deliveries following their Cesareans and I began thinking about it. It seemed like the impossible dream. Our first birth had been scary. I wasn't sure if I wanted to fight that fight or not. But the thought of being able to push the baby out, and all that that had meant to me before the first birth, kept running through my mind.

The United States is one of the few countries in which the "once a Cesarean . . ." dictum is followed. Studies from Great Britain, Ireland, and other countries have shown that vaginal deliveries in subsequent pregnancies are an accepted practice. Recent studies in the United States also show that vaginal delivery following a Cesarean is both feasible and safe. One, conducted at the University of Texas, followed 634 women who had one Cesarean delivery, through their next pregnancy. Of these, 526 were allowed a test of labor, and approximately half of these women experienced a successful vaginal delivery.[2] Some American doctors have reported much higher rates of success for vaginal delivery.

What about uterine rupture? This is the most often mentioned justification for repeat Cesarean delivery. Most doctors feel that the scar that resulted from the first surgery may not be able to withstand the stress of labor and delivery. The Texas study found that four of the women (three who had a trial of labor and one who had a planned repeat Cesarean) did experience some degree of rupture, although none of the women or the babies were seriously threatened as a result.

There is a vast difference between what most imagine happens in "uterine rupture" and what actually occurs. Part of the prob-

[2] Berkeley S. Merrill and C. E. Gibbs, "Planned Vaginal Delivery Following Cesarean Section," *Obstetrics and Gynecology* 52(1):50–52 (July 1978). The study examined 526 women who had one low cervical transverse Cesarean delivery. It showed that 49 per cent delivered vaginally, doing so with slightly less morbidity (problems) and a shorter hospital stay than 108 similar women who were not allowed a trial of labor. There was no difference in infant deaths or problems between the trial and the nontrial groups. An extensive bibliography on the subject of vaginal delivery following Cesarean birth is available from C/SEC Inc., 66 Christopher Road, Waltham, MA. 02154.

lem is the lack of a generally accepted definition of the word
"rupture." Rupture brings with it connotations of the uterus rapidly splitting apart, causing instant death to the baby and possibly
to the mother. This picture becomes reality only in extremely rare
circumstances. Most cases involve dehiscence (separation) of a
small portion of the scar from the first Cesarean. Very often this
separation appears to cause no problems during labor or delivery.
It occurs gradually during the course of pregnancy and causes no
discomfort. It is interesting that *Williams Obstetrics,* a standard
medical text, says that spontaneous rupture of the uterus "approxi-
mates or exceeds that of rupture of a Cesarean section scar and
today is probably more common than traumatic rupture."[3] Trans-
lated, this means a pregnant woman who has never had uterine
surgery is in as much danger of uterine rupture, as a result of her
pregnancy, as you are if you have a scar from a Cesarean delivery.

In light of all of this, why don't more doctors allow women at
least a trial of labor? Why don't more pregnant couples ask to attempt a vaginal delivery after Cesarean birth? Obviously the answers are complex.

Many doctors will agree that the chance of a uterine rupture is
indeed very small. They may tell you that while theoretically a
vaginal delivery is possible, it will probably not be an alternative
for you because of practical limitations. For instance, they may
say that vaginal delivery would not be safe unless you are 100 per
cent sure that an operating room and full staff would be immediately available during your entire labor. Even if your doctor is
willing, he or she may not be able to exercise this option in the
hospital where you deliver. It is the policy in some hospitals for
the obstetrics department to set guidelines on issues such as this,
which all physicians must follow. Another factor is the un-
willingness of many doctors to act in opposition to the prevalent
medical practice in their area. On an issue currently as controversial as this, their reticence increases. The malpractice crisis in
this country complicates the picture even further. A doctor who

[3] Jack A. Pritchard and Paul C. MacDonald, (eds.), *Williams Obstetrics*
(New York: Appleton-Century-Crofts, 1976).

allows you to deliver vaginally following a Cesarean could be courting a lawsuit, in the event something goes wrong. Selecting and monitoring a mother during an attempted vaginal delivery can be a complex procedure. If a serious problem does occur, your doctor could be held liable in the courts.

As parents you may come to the discussion with years of accumulated fears. It may be difficult even to bring up the subject with your doctor. One negative word from the obstetrician and you may find yourself ready to accept another Cesarean without further exploration of a vaginal delivery.

If you have such fears and your doctor is reluctant to consider vaginal delivery, you may never consider the issue in depth. Parents who question the doctor about the necessity of another Cesarean may encounter a "Who's in charge here?" response. Many couples still look at their doctor as an authority figure and they are unwilling or unable to question the judgment or opinion of a medical professional. (Some medical professionals do a lot to keep this authority-figure myth alive.) The decision to proceed with an attempt at a vaginal delivery should be a shared medical/ consumer responsibility, possibly involving a formalized agreement between you and your doctor.[4] If you decide you would like to attempt a vaginal delivery, there are many things to take into consideration.

*Finding a doctor who is supportive.* For many couples the first step is the biggest one. Once you have developed rapport with a doctor it may be difficult to seek other medical care, and this is just what you might be forced to do. It is possible to arrange consultations with doctors as you look for one who would be willing to let you attempt vaginal birth. This can be costly and time-consuming, and it requires energy that many pregnant couples do not have. You may never find a doctor who agrees. For one thing,

---

[4] Sample agreement:
We would like to have a trial of labor for the birth of our next baby. We have discussed the risks and benefits of this decision with you and understand both. We agree to be guided by your judgment during the labor and will agree to a Cesarean delivery if you deem it in the best interest of our child.

your doctor may have a sound medical reason for telling you a vaginal delivery is not advisable for you. You are certainly free to get a second opinion, but if this confirms the first you may want to begin planning a Cesarean delivery rather than continuing your search. Second, unless you live in an urban area affording choices within a reasonable distance of your home, your options may be very limited.

You may want to begin your search before you are pregnant a second time, so your entire pregnancy can be under one doctor's care. When and if you find a doctor who agrees, there are many questions you should discuss. It is important to know how your labor will be monitored and what conditions might make a second Cesarean necessary. You and your doctor will have time to plan for the best possible birth, be it vaginal or Cesarean.

*Finding a hospital where a trial of labor will be allowed.* Most hospitals allow each doctor to decide on an individual basis if a woman who has had a Cesarean delivery can attempt a vaginal birth. In others, the obstetrical unit sets policies that all doctors must follow. If your obstetrician has privileges (can practice medicine) at more than one hospital, he or she will guide you to the facility in your area that meets your needs, if one exists.

Sometimes the entire process must be done in reverse. You will have to locate a hospital that allows attempted vaginal deliveries and obtain a list of doctors who deliver there. Not everyone on the list will endorse this practice and you will have to search for a doctor who will be sympathetic to your request. You should inquire about the anesthesia department at the hospital also, since the facility you choose should probably have an anesthesiologist (a doctor who specializes in administering anesthesia) or a nurse anesthetist (a nurse trained in the use of anesthetic drugs) in the building twenty-four hours a day, seven days a week. Many hospitals do not have this coverage but rather have an anesthesiologist or anesthetist within fifteen minutes of the hospital.

*Good medical records from your first Cesarean.* You will have to be able to provide your obstetrician with complete information on your Cesarean delivery. This must include the kind of uterine scar you have and whether any medical complications, especially infections, followed your delivery. Your doctor will need to understand as much as possible about your medical history to make a valid judgment about the advisability of vaginal delivery for you.

*The reason for your first Cesarean is no longer present.* Many Cesareans are now done for reasons particular to a pregnancy. A baby in the breech position (feet or buttocks first) or one in fetal distress usually has nothing to do with the mother's anatomy or medical condition, and therefore these problems would not predictably occur in future pregnancies. It would be unusual to have a second breech baby or another child go into severe fetal distress, although it is possible. Even CPD cephalo-pelvic disproportion is no longer considered an absolute indication for a second Cesarean delivery. Many women are able to vaginally deliver an even larger baby in a second pregnancy.

*A willingness to accept another Cesarean delivery if necessary.* Well over half of the women who are allowed a trial of labor in the United States do have vaginal deliveries. For those who don't, it may be difficult to hope once again for a vaginal birth and instead have to physically and emotionally deal with a second Cesarean delivery.

This certainly doesn't mean you shouldn't try if you want to and your doctor agrees. It is best if you plan ahead so that either mode of delivery will be a good one. This includes discussing with your doctor what medical conditions would indicate that another Cesarean was necessary. Also talk over the kinds of anesthesia that are available in your area and decide what type you prefer. If you would like to be together for either a vaginal or a Cesarean birth, plan for this too.

My first pregnancy had produced a fantastic 8 pound boy. He was a Cesarean baby because he was breech. When I became pregnant again, I found that I was spending a lot of time thinking about trying a vaginal delivery. I hesitated for a long time before I approached my doctor about the possibilities. I wouldn't say she jumped up and down in glee at the prospect, but she did, after many discussions, agree to let me try.

The months leading up to the delivery seemed to drag on forever. The closer my due date came, the more questions I had about what I was doing. Most of the time, I only remembered the negative things I had read or heard about vaginal delivery after a Cesarean. But I wanted to do this so much that I just had to hang in there. I finally went into labor about three days after my due date and off to the hospital we went. The hospital staff really kept track of how I was doing. The further my labor progressed, the closer they watched me! I made it through transition and they wheeled me down to the delivery room. We were so close I could hardly concentrate on what I was supposed to be doing. My husband joined me and we *pushed that baby out*. It was fantastic. It was incredible. It was exactly what I had hoped it would be and even more.

## CEPHALO-PELVIC DISPROPORTION (CPD a spatial problem between mother and baby)

More primary (first) Cesarean deliveries are done because of cephalo-pelvic disproportion than for any other reason. Often the word "relative" is placed before cephalo-pelvic disproportion, and it is very important. When the size of your pelvis is compared with the size of your baby's head, the doctor may decide that passage through the vaginal canal might take a toll on one or both of you. Often this spatial problem is compounded by the baby's position in your uterus. If the baby's head is not flexed tightly against his chest and the presenting part (the part that would pass through the birth canal first) is his brow, or if his head has not rotated and he is looking up instead of down, he will need even more room than usual to pass safely through your pelvic opening. The reason "relative" is central to your delivery is that if your baby were smaller and in a slightly different position, or if your pelvic measurements were slightly larger, then a vaginal delivery might have been possible. There are a few women who have an anatomical problem called a severely contracted pelvis, which so limits the space available to the baby that a vaginal delivery is simply out of the question.

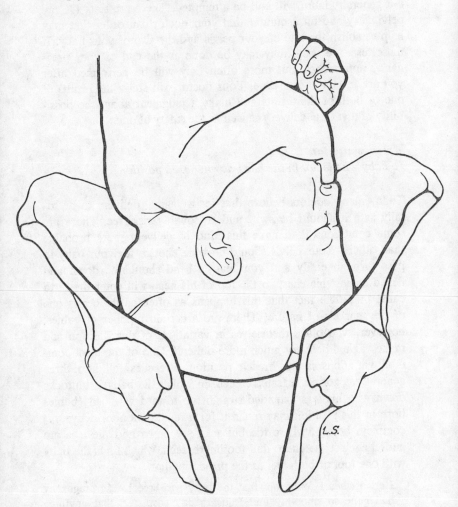

*Cephalo-pelvic Disproportion*   The baby's head is too large to pass safely through the mother's pelvis.

It is usually difficult for the doctor to determine the extent of disproportion before you are in labor. In a few cases, your obstetrician may be fairly certain that a Cesarean will be necessary, but generally labor will still be attempted. There are tests (X ray pelvimetry and ultrasound[5]) that your doctor can order that may help establish the size of your pelvis and the size of your baby. If these tests are used, they may be done as the end of your pregnancy approaches, but more often they will be performed after you are in labor for a time. Your doctor will study the results of one or both of these tests and make a judgment about the possibility of a vaginal delivery as well as the safety of one.

## *Malpresentation*
*(a baby who is not in the head-down, flexed position)*

Today many doctors believe that for a vaginal delivery to be totally safe it should be swift and reasonably risk-free. There are some conditions that make this kind of delivery more probable than others. Your pelvis should be wide enough for your baby to pass through easily and your baby's head should be down and flexed against his chest so the top of his head will enter the birth canal first. The fact that this happens as often as it does is one of the marvels of nature! There are a certain number of babies, however, who place themselves in variations of this position and make vaginal delivery much more difficult. One of the most common variations is the breech position. Breeches fall into three general categories: a frank breech, in which the baby is buttocks down with his legs extended straight up toward his head (babies born in this position may retain it for a few hours after delivery); complete breech, where the buttocks are down and the legs are curled against the chest; and footling breech, which finds the baby with one foot or both feet as the presenting part.

I cried when I found out that the baby was breech. My pregnancy had gone so smoothly and I just hadn't suspected that anything

---

[5] All the tests mentioned in this chapter are discussed in detail in Chapter Three.

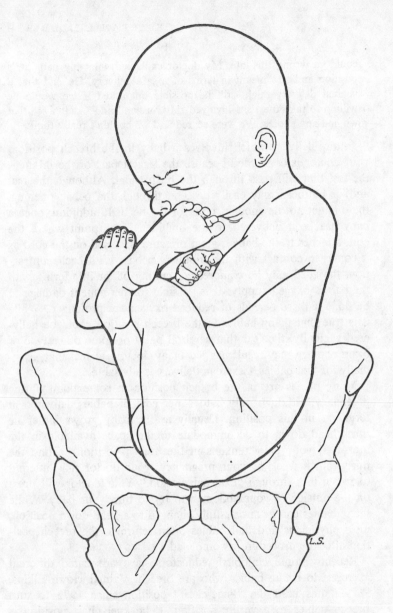

*Frank Breech*   This illustration shows the baby in a frank breech position. The baby's buttocks would be the first part to pass through the pelvis.

could go wrong this late. My doctor explained what my daughter's position and size meant in terms of a safe delivery. He said that a vaginal delivery might still be possible but asked if we would be willing to take the risks involved. My husband and I didn't see that we had any choice. We were scared and we couldn't really think.

In any delivery which involves a baby in the breech position, your doctor is concerned because the largest part of the infant is the last that will pass through the birth canal. Although the feet and/or buttocks may easily descend through the pelvic opening, there might not be enough room for the head. In addition, once a baby has been delivered to the umbilicus (the point where the cord attaches to the baby), great pressure is placed on the cord as it comes in contact with the mother's pelvis. With each contraction, the cord may be compressed, cutting off or interfering with the baby's oxygen supply. It is possible for permanent damage to be done if these periods of reduced oxygen are prolonged. While it is true that many babies in the breech position could be delivered vaginally, the fear that cerebral palsy or some other type of brain damage may result has led many doctors to feel that, especially for first babies, Cesarean delivery is advisable.

Many babies are in the breech position at some point during pregnancy, although only 3 to 4 per cent of babies delivered at term are in this position. Usually as the baby grows larger he turns head down to accommodate to the space available in the uterus. If your baby remains in the breech position beyond the thirty-fourth week of your pregnancy, your doctor may attempt to rotate him through "external version." Your doctor will press on the outside of your abdomen to try to turn your baby. While many babies can be successfully changed to a head-down position, most physicians find that babies often return to the breech position after the procedure is completed.

Recently some childbirth educators have advocated different exercises to rotate babies who are breech. Valmai Howe Elkins, R.P.T., has used the "knee-chest" position since 1973 to turn breech babies to a vertex position. (The knee-chest position is taught in most childbirth preparation classes as an aid in relieving pressure discomfort in the lower back and abdomen during pregnancy.) Seventy-one women, whose babies were determined to be in the breech position from the thirty-seventh week of pregnancy on, followed the procedure. Sixty-five of those babies turned from breech to vertex and all of these were normal vaginal births. The six babies who remained breech were all born by Cesarean. Of these babies, two had a low-lying placenta, two had an unusually short umbilical cord and one mother had a bicornuate (two-chambered) uterus.

Ms. Elkins found in most cases that fifteen minutes of the "knee-chest" position repeated every two hours of waking time for five days produced the results reported above. Two thirds of those babies who turned were diagnosed vertex after five days' use of the position. The remainder turned following a repetition of the procedure. All seventy-one women were enrolled in Elkins' childbirth education classes and were taught the position with particular attention to correct positioning of hips, back, and knees. Head and shoulder position varied slightly according to comfort. Each woman had her doctor's approval for use of the procedure. Elkins feels strongly that this procedure should be supervised by a doctor or a childbirth educator as it can not only be extremely uncomfortable but can actually produce or aggravate backache if done incorrectly. She also notes that it is not recommended for a footling breech presentation.

Another position some babies elect in the uterus is termed a transverse lie. In this position, the baby is stretched across the uterus at a forty-five-degree angle to the mother's spinal column. Generally the baby's shoulder is the presenting part. If a vaginal delivery were attempted, the shoulder would be forced into the pelvic opening first, blocking passage of the rest of the baby's body. This position occurs rarely, but when it does, a Cesarean delivery is almost always necessary.

Other malpresentations include brow presentations in which the baby's head is not flexed against the chest; face presentations, where the baby's head is extended and the face is forced to enter the birth canal first; or a sincipital (the upper half of the skull) position, where the large fontanel (soft spot) of the head descends first. These conditions alone do not usually make a Cesarean delivery necessary. Often they occur with some other factor, such as fetal distress or a nonprogressive labor, and the combination may lead to a Cesarean.

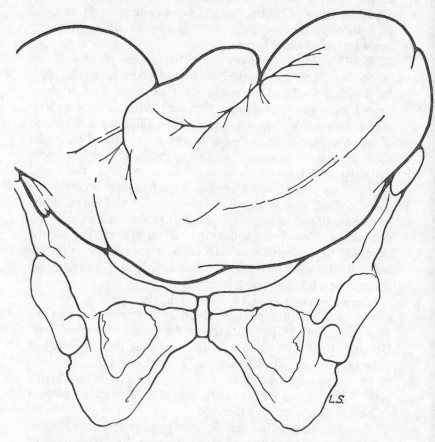

*Transverse Lie* The baby is stretched from left to right across the mother's uterus. Usually the shoulder descends first and blocks the passage of the rest of the baby.

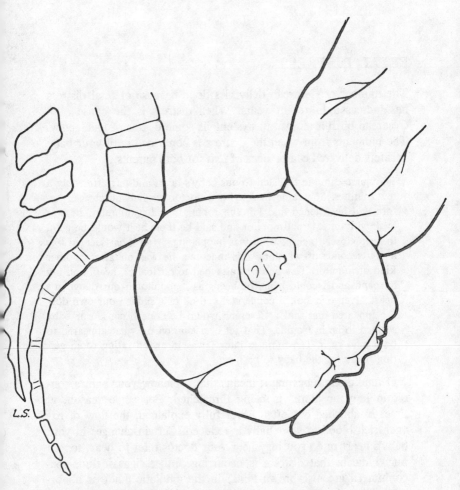

*Brow Presentation* The baby's head is not flexed down on the chest, so the largest diameter of the head would be forced to pass through the pelvis first.

## FETAL DISTRESS

The number of Cesarean deliveries done because of fetal distress has increased in recent years. When distress is the cause of a Cesarean birth it almost always entails some degree of emergency. The moments from when the distress is confirmed until your baby is safely delivered can be ones of fear for both parents.

> The nurse came in to listen to our baby's heart and left after only a few minutes. She came back with a doctor we had never seen before and he listened and left the room. In a few minutes, he was back with an external monitor and said he thought it would be good to keep closer track of what was happening. After what seemed like a few seconds of watching this machine, he was off after another kind of monitor. This one was attached to our baby's head, and my husband and I could hear the beeps as it monitored our daughter's heart. Everyone looked concerned and all of a sudden our own doctor appeared and said a Cesarean would be done because our baby seemed to be in trouble. That set everyone off on what appeared to be a mad rush. Ten minutes later I was in an operating room getting ready for the baby to be born.

If fetal distress occurs, it means that somehow your baby's condition in your uterus is being threatened. For some reason, at times established but often never fully explained, the flow of oxygen-rich blood to your baby is reduced. Certain changes in your baby's heart rate (you may hear your doctor refer to heart tones) may indicate that distress is occurring. Other signs include meconium (a greenish-brown fluid) in the amniotic fluid, or abnormally vigorous movements by the baby. An additional indicator of distress is an abnormality in the pH in blood samples taken from your baby's scalp. pH measures the acidity or alkalinity of your baby's blood; if the pH is abnormal, it indicates that distress is indeed occurring.

Your baby's heartbeat pattern changes during the course of

labor, just as yours does as you undergo different types of activity during the day. Contractions can cause slight compressions of the cord or mild pressure on your baby's head, which result in a change in heartbeats. This is a normal part of labor. Your doctor will be concerned if your baby's heart rate remains slow as a contraction subsides and continues to be slow during the time between contractions. Extreme variations in heart rate or a very rapid rate also mean that further investigation should be done.

## PREMATURE or PROLONGED RUPTURE OF THE MEMBRANES

I got up about three o'clock in the morning because I felt a sudden gush of water. After my third trip to the bathroom, my husband asked me what was going on. I said that I thought my membranes had ruptured. He said that he thought I should know one way or the other. We had just finished six weeks of childbirth classes and we were supposed to know these things. I wasn't in labor. I wasn't even uncomfortable. I was just dripping. I called the doctor, embarrassed to be making that 3:00 A.M. phone call. He said to wait twenty-four hours and then come to the hospital if labor hadn't brought me there sooner. For a whole day my husband and I stared at my abdomen, waiting for something to happen. It never did.

Usually if your membranes rupture before labor begins (something that happens in about 10 per cent of all pregnancies), labor will start within approximately twenty-four hours. Once your membranes have ruptured, your baby is exposed to the danger of infection, since his protective sac has been broken. Even if antibiotics are given to the mother, they do not reduce the risk to the baby. Approximately 3 to 5 per cent of the women whose membranes rupture at term do not go into labor within twenty-four hours, the period that most doctors feel it is safe to wait. If this time goes by and there are no signs of labor, most doctors will try to induce labor. You will be given an oxytocic drug (a synthetic hormone that stimulates contractions) by intravenous infusion (IV). There is a good chance that labor will begin and that you will deliver vaginally. If this does not happen, the baby still must be delivered, and a Cesarean will be necessary.

# FAILURE TO PROGRESS—UTERINE INERTIA OR DYSFUNCTION

I had been in labor for twelve hours and the baby just wouldn't be born. I was really getting depressed and began to feel as though I might fall apart. My doctor ordered X rays. I was given Pitocin. Nothing seemed to help, and my doctor said he thought a Cesarean would be necessary. I really didn't care just then. I was tired and discouraged and I wanted it all to end. Afterward I kept wondering if I had done something wrong. Perhaps if I had been stronger or tried a little harder, I could have had a vaginal delivery.

Labor can begin with all the signs you have learned to expect, then seem to go on and on without producing a baby. Sometimes contractions start out strong and regular, then become weak and erratic. Contractions can feel very strong and still your cervix does not open or your baby's head doesn't drop into the birth canal. When this happens, it is often a natural protection against a pelvis that is smaller than usual or a baby who is rather large or in an abnormal position. Your uterus may slow down rather than continuing to force your baby through a pelvic opening that is just not big enough. Other things that can affect the kind of contractions you have are anxiety, exhaustion, multiple births, and many previous deliveries.

Although every woman's labor is different, a unifying characteristic of all labor is progression. After studying the progress of hundreds of normal labors, various graphs or timelines have been established that show the usual relationship between the time in labor, the amount of dilation of the cervix, and the descent of the baby's head into the pelvis. (One you may hear referred to is the

Friedman Curve.) Your doctor may compare your labor to these guides, and if any one stage does become prolonged, he will use this as an indication that further investigation is needed.

Steps may be taken to stimulate your labor. You may be given oxytocin, to stimulate contractions. You may be encouraged to change position in bed or to get up and walk for a while. Most women are kept on their backs during labor. Recent research has shown that this has few advantages.[6] Standing, squatting, and walking tend to produce stronger and more efficient labor contractions as well as to shorten labor and make the mother more comfortable. If your doctor feels that tension may be slowing your labor, you might be offered a mild tranquilizer. Although you may have wished for an unmedicated birth, sometimes a small dose of medication may be just what is needed to allow your labor to progress. If none of these attempts stimulates labor a Cesarean delivery may be recommended, for an overly-long labor can involve risks for your baby as well as be a physical and emotional drain on you.

Sometimes women feel their doctors want to hasten labor for less than medical reasons (a backlog of office patients or an approaching weekend). Although this can happen in rare instances, most often the decision to perform a Cesarean is based on your doctor's concern for your baby and for you.

## HEMORRHAGE-PLACENTA PREVIA AND ABRUPTIO PLACENTA

Your baby receives oxygen and nutrients from you through the placenta. When the placenta attaches to the wall of your uterus,

[6] Roberto Calderyo-Barcia, M.D., "The Influence of Maternal Position on Time of Spontaneous Rupture of the Membranes, Progress of Labor, and Fetal Head Compression," *Birth and the Family Journal,* Vol. 6, No. 1 (Spring 1979), pp. 7–15.

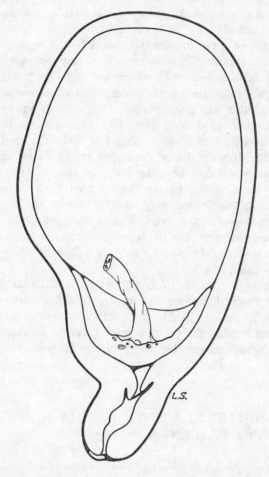

*Placenta Previa* The placenta has attached over the vaginal opening and it would pass through the birth canal before the baby.

ideally it does so near the top. Sometimes it adheres very low in your uterus, where the lining is less nourishing and the blood supply is not as adequate. Then the placenta spreads out over a larger surface to insure access to enough of your blood supply. In doing so, it may cover all, part of, or just the rim of your cervix. Sometimes it does not come in contact with your cervix at all until you are in labor and your cervix begins to dilate (open). There are many dangers in this situation, including maternal hemorrhage, obstruction of your baby's passage through the birth canal, and separation of the placenta during labor.

Often a mother with a placenta previa will experience bleeding during the last three months of pregnancy. If bleeding stops or decreases and time permits, your doctor will probably do some tests to see how well your baby would do if delivered. (Two tests used are ultrasound and amniocentesis.) Once your doctor feels your baby will survive if delivered, a Cesarean will be done. Not every case of placenta previa ends with a Cesarean delivery, though most do. If the placenta is not blocking your cervix, a vaginal delivery may be possible.

Another type of uterine hemorrhage is caused by the early separation of the placenta from your uterine wall. This is called abruptio placenta. Often the separation does not become apparent until just before or during labor, although it may have begun sometime previously. Again, there is danger that your baby's oxygen supply may be interrupted, and delivery usually must occur quickly. How quickly depends on the amount of separation that has taken place, since oxygen and carbon dioxide can be transferred in adequate amounts across a partially detached placenta.

Both placenta previa and abruptio placenta are dangerous for mother and baby. Cesarean delivery has been found a safe way to minimize some of the risks involved.

When tests showed that the placenta was unusually low in the uterus and covered the cervix, I was told to plan on a Cesarean. Our first reaction to the news was keen disappointment. My husband was especially disappointed, since he wouldn't be allowed in the operating room. Having my baby without him there made childbirth look like a lonely ordeal for me instead of an exciting adventure for both of us. I thought I would be a slab of meat someone would cut up, a far cry from my vision of an "awake and aware" childbirth.

Since there was danger of losing my baby, I was confined to bed for the last two months of my pregnancy. After all those weeks of anxious waiting, how we had our baby became increasingly unimportant. We just wanted a healthy baby any way we could. When the baby was finally big enough to have a good chance for survival even if he came early, our thankfulness for our child's continuing life overshadowed any fear or anxiety we might have had.

## CORD ACCIDENTS

Your baby is dependent on the oxygen supply that flows from your body through the placenta and through a cord that connects the placenta to your baby. Usually this umbilical cord is about two feet long, and it should float freely in your uterus. Sometimes the cord wraps around part of your baby's body or enters the birth canal first. If it becomes twisted around your baby, it can interfere with the infant's circulation, although many babies are safely delivered vaginally with the cord wrapped around their necks. If the cord prolapses (enters the birth canal first), however, it can be very serious. With each contraction, the cord is squeezed between your baby's head and your pelvis, leaving your baby momentarily without oxygen. A prolapsed cord almost always means an emergency Cesarean delivery.

## PREMATURITY

The word "premature" can be used to describe a variety of circumstances. It can mean a baby who weighs less than 5½ pounds or one who is delivered before the thirty-eighth week of pregnancy. "Premature" can describe babies with low birth weights who are mature in every other way. (These babies are also called "small for dates.") It can be used to describe a baby who weighs more than 5½ pounds but has immature vital organs such as the heart, liver, kidneys, and lungs.

A premature baby may not be large enough or sufficiently mature to withstand labor or life outside the uterus as well as a mature, full-sized infant. Whether labor happens spontaneously or is induced, the premature infant's system may be exposed to more stress than it can tolerate. Premature labors are usually carefully monitored and, if distress occurs that cannot be corrected, a Cesarean delivery will be done for your baby's well being.

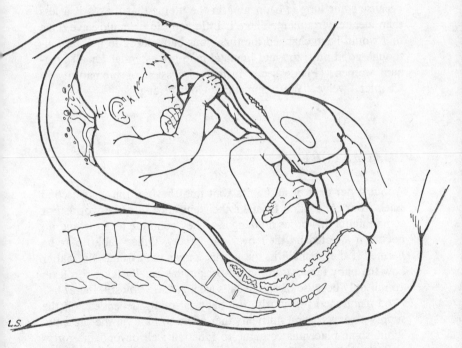

*Prolapsed Cord* The baby's cord has prolapsed or become wedged between the baby and the pelvic opening. With each contraction the cord is further compressed and the baby's oxygen supply is interrupted to some degree.

I thought I was due in the middle of May. Here it was the first week of April and I was in labor. All I could think was, "Oh, no, not yet. The poor baby doesn't have enough clothes, a place to sleep, or even a diaper." I was sure they would send me home from the hospital and tell me it was all a mistake.

No obvious reason can be found to explain about 60 per cent of the premature births that occur. Often women blame themselves for their baby's early arrival and go through a list of "ifs." "If I hadn't played tennis" or "if I hadn't gone grocery shopping" are examples of the kind of thoughts that can follow a premature birth. Many doctors feel that a baby is born prematurely because something is happening in the uterus that makes it a less than ideal environment. There is little you did or could have done that would have changed the time your baby chose to be born, although good nutrition and prenatal care are essential for all pregnant women. (Please see a further discussion of prematurity in Chapter Twelve, "When Something Goes Wrong.")

## POSTMATURITY

About 4 per cent of all babies wait until beyond the forty-second week from conception to make their entrance into the world. For some infants this poses no dangers. They continue to grow and do not seem affected by their overly-long stay. Other babies may be harmed if they remain in the uterus longer than usual. No matter how the baby fares, a prolonged pregnancy usually takes a toll on you, if only because of phone calls asking, "Are you still there?"

As mentioned previously, the baby is totally dependent on the supply of oxygen and nutrients that come to him via the placenta. While some placentas continue to function well beyond the forty-second week, many begin to slow down or age. Your baby may actually begin to lose weight and become malnourished. If your baby shows no sign of arriving two weeks after your estimated due date, the situation warrants investigation. There are tests that your doctor can order. (Ultrasound, amniocentesis, and estriols are commonly used.) If any of these show that your baby may be in danger, you will probably be asked to come into the hospital for an attempted induction of labor. There are times when induction does not stimulate sustained, effective labor and a Cesarean delivery is necessary.

## MULTIPLE BIRTHS

When a Cesarean delivery is necessary for a multiple birth (twins, triplets, etc.), it is usually because one or more of the babies is in an abnormal position. Multiple babies are usually smaller than those born singly, so are freer to move about and assume a wide variety of positions in the uterus.

## ADVANCED MATERNAL AGE

As more women wait to begin their families until after the age of thirty or thirty-five, concern about the relationship of age and method of delivery continues to surface. Although there used to be some sentiment that once a woman reached her mid-thirties her body was no longer capable of vaginal delivery, this is no longer thought to be the case. It is true that the older the woman, the greater the chance that a medical problem may be present (such as diabetes or hypertension) that might make a Cesarean necessary. However, age in itself is not the determining factor, especially now that women take a much greater interest in nutrition and exercise programs. Certainly a woman who is thirty-five or older is perfectly able to deliver a healthy child. However, your age may have some bearing on how your baby is delivered. Recent research indicates that the Cesarean rate for women delivering their first baby after their mid-thirties greatly exceeds the rate for younger women. All of the reasons for this increase have not been identified, but one consideration is the number of childbearing years available to the "older mother." Your doctor may advocate a Cesarean delivery for you that he or she might not feel was as necessary for a younger woman.

## MATERNAL MEDICAL CONDITIONS

There are a number of medical conditions that can affect the course of your pregnancy. Although they are quite different for the mother, they are similar in that they may pose a threat to your baby, usually even before labor begins. When one of these conditions is present, it is often desirable for your' baby to be delivered before your actual due date. Usually your doctor will try to induce labor, but if this is not successful, a Cesarean delivery will be necessary.

### Diabetes

The number of childbearing women who have diabetes has increased over the past fifty years. Many things explain this increase, including a longer life expectancy for anyone with diabetes because of advances in medical care and improved methods for early diagnosis of this disease. Diabetes, which occurs in about 2 per cent of all pregnancies, is characterized by an imbalance in the body between sugar and the hormone insulin, which is responsible for processing sugar. If insulin is not present in sufficient amounts, the sugar builds up in the blood and begins to be cleared by the kidneys.

Pregnancy can cause changes in diabetes. The amount of insulin being taken must be monitored very closely and sometimes frequently changed. A diabetic mother must watch her diet carefully, guard against infection, and have regular tests to monitor the amount of sugar in blood and urine. Toxemia (see following discussion) occurs more frequently in pregnant women with diabetes than in those without this disease.

The baby can also be affected by the diabetes. Babies of diabetic mothers tend to be larger than the norm and show a higher incidence of respiratory distress syndrome (RDS, a disease of newborns characterized by immature lungs). Diabetic women face a higher risk of stillbirth if their pregnancy goes to full term. Because of this, the doctor will usually order some tests of fetal maturity (ultrasound and amniocentesis) and then try to induce labor around the thirty-seventh or thirty-eighth week of pregnancy. Unless the baby's head has dropped into your pelvis and your cervix has begun to soften and dilate, there is little chance that labor will successfully be stimulated. A Cesarean delivery would then be done to minimize the risk for both you and your baby.

> All the time I was growing up I wondered if I would be able to have a baby since I was a diabetic. I lived with a lot of fear and uncertainty during the first months of my pregnancy. My doctor was very supportive. She kept saying I could do it. When she said the baby would probably have to be a Cesarean delivery, it really didn't matter a bit to me. I wanted this baby so very, very much. Anything that could be done to give it to me was just fine.

Some women develop symptoms of diabetes only when they are pregnant. This type of diabetes is called gestational or "Class A" diabetes. It is usually detected during a prenatal office visit. Although gestational diabetics must watch their diets carefully and have frequent tests to monitor sugar levels in blood and urine, most pregnancies proceed normally. Usually all signs of diabetes end with the pregnancy, although they may recur with future children.

## Toxemia of Pregnancy

The term "toxemia" is used to describe a trio of findings, including high blood pressure, protein in the urine, and overall retention of fluids resulting in swelling of greater than normal amounts. It is not understood why toxemia occurs, but it continues to be one of the most dangerous conditions of pregnancy. The disease can range from very mild to severe.

Milder forms of toxemia can sometimes be brought under control through the use of medication, diet control, and bed rest. Management of toxemia has undergone some changes. Doctors recognize that bed rest is currently the most effective way of controlling the disease and avoiding the complications that diuretics and salt-free diets may involve. Your doctor will probably advise tests for fetal maturity and attempt to induce labor when your baby appears ready to be born. If the toxemia is not severe and if your baby is not mature enough, your pregnancy will continue for a while longer.

There are two forms of severe toxemia: severe pre-eclampsia and eclampsia. Severe pre-eclampsia usually occurs during the last twenty weeks of pregnancy. It can be signaled by sudden excessive weight gain, protein in the urine, and severe swelling of the feet and legs. Increasing hypertension (high blood pressure) is the most consistent sign that severe pre-eclampsia may be beginning. Eclampsia has the signs of severe pre-eclampsia plus convulsions and/or coma. Many times a premature baby of a mother with severe toxemia fares better in an intensive care nursery than he would have had the pregnancy continued.

Good prenatal care usually will detect signs of toxemia. If the disease is detected early enough, your doctor may have time to begin appropriate management to control the disease sufficiently so the outlook for you and your baby is improved.

### Rh Disease (Erythroblastosis Fetalis)

Cesarean delivery is certainly not indicated simply because a woman has Rh-negative blood. It is becoming increasingly uncommon for difficulties to arise in pregnancies involving Rh-negative women, although problems do occur on occasion. Sometimes an Rh-negative woman has difficulties because, either during pregnancy or following a transfusion of Rh-positive blood, antibodies formed in her blood. The antibodies she develops can pass through the placenta and attack the red blood cells of the baby. The infant must then produce additional red blood cells, but in time production loses out to destruction, and the baby may develop a severe fetal anemia called erythroblastosis fetalis.

Erythroblastosis fetalis is disappearing now that most Rh-negative women who deliver Rh-positive babies are given the drug RhoGAM within seventy-two hours of the birth. However, there continue to be a few women who are not given this injection or who are sensitized through some other means. When this happens, various tests are used to follow the pregnancy closely. If it appears that your baby is becoming anemic or jaundiced and is mature enough to survive outside of your uterus, you will be asked to come to the hospital and an induction of labor will be attempted. If labor cannot be sustained, a Cesarean delivery will be done. If the tests show that your baby is anemic but is not mature enough to be born, it is now possible to give the infant blood transfusions while he is still in your uterus.

### High Blood Pressure (Chronic Hypertension)
Women who suffer from high blood pressure may experience constriction of their blood vessels, which can cause problems during pregnancy. The baby receives its supply of oxygen and needed nutrients from the mother's blood through the placenta. If the mother's system cannot supply the uterus with the normal amount of blood, the baby may be endangered, especially during labor.

Usually good prenatal care is all that is needed for women with mild or moderate hypertension, although there should be frequent checks for toxemia, and the baby's progress should be closely watched. Women with more severe high blood pressure must be carefully monitored during their pregnancy. Often, for the sake of the baby, a Cesarean delivery will be advised.

### Heart Disease
Heart disease is not in itself an indication for a Cesarean delivery. An increasing number of women who have had cardiac surgery reach childbearing age and have vaginal deliveries. Each case must, of course, be judged individually, but current thought seems

to be that women with heart disease can manage labor and vaginal deliveries very well.

### Renal or Kidney Disease

The urinary system undergoes changes during pregnancy. It must be able to handle increased reabsorption of salt and water as well as to maintain the overall fluid balance in the body. A woman who suffers from kidney disease may experience difficulties during pregnancy as a result of these added demands on her system. Also, kidney or renal disease is often accompanied by high blood pressure and the risks discussed above if that disease is present.

### Fibroid Tumors

These are benign (noncancerous) tumors found on or within the uterine wall. Most women who have this type of tumor deliver vaginally. Occasionally fibroid tumors may grow, because of hormones produced during pregnancy, and interfere with labor and delivery. Usually the tumors are not removed since, even if a Cesarean becomes necessary, the growth subsides, and once again they become harmless with the end of pregnancy.

### Herpes Infection

This is a viral disease that has been found with increasing frequency in pregnant women over the last few years. Much like the mouth can develop fever blisters or cold sores, the vaginal area can harbor a similar kind of virus. This virus produces blisters on the vaginal walls and cervix. It was formerly thought that babies were protected from this infection by antibodies transferred through the placenta. It is now known that, if the baby is born vaginally and open sores are present, widespread infection can occur that can even result in the death of the baby. A Cesarean delivery will protect the baby from this risk if performed within four hours of rupture of the membranes.

### Previous Uterine Surgery

Women who have had surgery that involved either their uterus or vaginal tract will be carefully evaluated by their doctor to see if a vaginal delivery is possible. The major concern is the strength of the scar or scars that resulted from the previous surgery. If the scar is large, or if there is any danger of rupture, a Cesarean delivery will be advisable.

# THREE

# Tests Used During Pregnancy and Delivery

Your pregnancy may be very uneventful and routine prenatal visits will be the only contact you have with your doctor or with medical procedures. On the other hand, you may find that one or more tests will be used to follow your progress, especially if you are scheduled to have a Cesarean delivery. There are also tests and procedures that may be used while you are in labor, and you should be familiar with these as well.

Many of these tests are relatively new, and some remain controversial. Very often, those who hold differing opinions either completely support or totally reject a specific test for the sake of their argument rather than attempt to find a balance between the known benefits and the unknown risks. Others argue that while tests may be justified in individual cases, too often they become standard medical procedure during all pregnancies. With strong feelings on both sides, problems of communication continue to grow between health care professionals, who may feel that their judgment is implicitly questioned when parents wish to discuss their advice, and consumers, who are faced with dramatic accounts of suspected risks involved in accepting this same advice.

As the use of technology in childbirth grows, concern increases. There is a fear that many normal variations in pregnancy or delivery are now considered complications that can only be corrected by sophisticated medical intervention. We have entered what some perceive as a technological race in obstetrical care. Especially in areas where there is more than one facility, doctors and hospitals may vie to be the "first on their block" to buy a new machine or implement a new procedure. This is often aggravated by consumers who judge a medical facility on the basis of the latest machines it owns.

There is an eagerness among some medical professionals and laypeople to embrace new tests and procedures out of a genuine concern to improve care. However, there are some professionals and laypeople who feel that such innovations are accepted before adequate studies on the risks and benefits have been done. On the other hand, health care professionals wonder how long a machine or a drug is "new" and how procedures that not only prevent problems at birth but also may prevent deaths can be questioned. To all of this, we must add the fact that suits have been filed and judgments won by parents against doctors because available tests were not used to determine the maturity or health of their baby.

What should be remembered is that all of these tests are tools to be used judiciously by your physician. There are tests that were initially developed for very specific complications of pregnancy that are now routinely used for almost all women. You have the right to know why any test will be used during your pregnancy. You also have the right to know the possible risks associated with the procedures that might be used. Some of the responsibility for gathering such information rests with you. Periodicals, books, childbirth classes, and thorough discussions with your doctor will help you understand how a particular test can be of benefit to you. Also, you may refuse to accept any test or procedure after considering the alternatives that could result from this refusal. Before you make your decision, make sure you completely understand why your doctor thinks a certain procedure or test is necessary, and consider your responsibility for the health of your baby.

# ELECTRONIC FETAL MONITORS

### What Happens

There are two types of electronic fetal monitors (EFMs) now widely in use.

The *external monitor* consists of two bands or belts, sometimes joined as one, which are strapped around your abdomen. One belt measures uterine contractions, and the other the baby's heart rate and general heart pattern. The bands are attached to a recording device, which continuously graphs the information. This type of monitor is painless for both mother and baby and is easily attached. You must remain in one position, usually on your back, for it to record accurately. If the picture given by the external monitor is positive, it is a generally reliable tool. If it shows some abnormalities, however, usually an internal monitor will replace it, since troublesome readings are often inaccurate.

To prepare for *internal monitoring,* your membranes (sac of water) must be broken if they have not already ruptured. An electrode is then attached directly to your baby's scalp with a tiny spiral-shaped needle. If your baby is born with hair, you probably won't notice this mark. If you can see it, it will be a tiny scab, which will disappear in a few days. A pressure catheter (a thin tube) will be inserted into your uterus to measure the strength of your contractions. It is fairly simple to complete both steps and should take only a few minutes. You may find that relaxation breathing patterns taught in childbirth preparation classes are helpful while the procedure is being completed.

Monitors audibly reproduce your baby's heart rate, as well as providing a graph of the baby's heart pattern and your contractions. Most machines have a control that adjusts the sound portion. Feel free to ask someone to turn this down if it bothers you. Greater movement is possible with internal monitoring than with an external monitor, since motion does not affect the accuracy of the reading. However, the actual distance you can go is limited by the length of the wires. The wires can come loose as you move. It is not catastrophic if this happens, since they can be easily reattached, but it may give you a momentary start if the sound from the machine suddenly stops. Sometimes the staff may be willing to unhook briefly the wires so that you can move around or go to the bathroom.

## Why

Listening to a baby's heart provides the doctor with extremely valuable information about how the baby is withstanding the stress of labor. Monitoring during labor has gone on for many years. Until fairly recently, it was done primarily by a nurse using a special stethoscope called a fetoscope. Now many hospitals use some type of electronic fetal monitor for all women in labor.

## Considerations

As the use of electronic fetal monitors continues to grow, the controversy surrounding their use increases also. Should all women be electronically monitored during labor? Are monitors being used as one tool among many available to evaluate labor, or is an abnormal monitor reading accepted as sufficient reason for an immediate Cesarean delivery without further investigation?

In many hospitals external monitoring is now used during all labors. Some routinely use internal monitoring. Although opinion seems to be growing to support the use of EFMs in high-risk pregnancies, there is a diversity of opinion on the benefits to be gained in using these machines for all labors. A recent task force of the National Institute of Child Health and Human Development listed specific situations which would be considered high risk.[1] These include: low birth weight, prematurity, postmaturity,

[1] William A. Check, "Electronic Fetal Monitoring: How Necessary?" *Journal of American Medical Association,* Vol. 241, No. 17 (Apr. 27, 1979), p. 1,772. This article reports the findings of a recent National Institute of Child Health and Human Development Task Force. A full report of the committee can be obtained by writing: NICHHD, Building 31, Room 2A34, Bethesda, Md. 20014.

medical complications of pregnancy (such as diabetes or high blood pressure), meconium in the amniotic fluid, oxytocin used in labor, low-risk women whose actual labor does not proceed routinely, and abnormal fetal heart rate on auscultation (nurse listening with a fetoscope). About one quarter of all pregnancies would be included if these conditions were the only ones in which an electronic monitor were used.

Two recent studies explored what occurred while continuous electronic monitoring was used.[2] Both found that mothers and babies fared equally well whether electronic monitoring was used or whether they were intermittently monitored by a nurse. Both also found that neither beneficial nor harmful effects of continuous fetal heart monitors could be validated. There was a one-to-one relationship between nurse and mother for those women who labored without an electronic monitor. The nurse listened to the baby's heartbeat every fifteen minutes in the first stage of labor and more frequently as labor progressed. Measurements were made either during or within thirty seconds of a labor contraction. Realistically, this type of care is available in only selected maternity facilities. It is much more usual for a nurse to have care of a number of women and to check each at longer intervals. Some women now hire private nurses so they can be assured of one-to-one care during their labor, especially if they would prefer not to be electronically monitored. Other hospitals are establishing birthing centers that provide a well-trained staff to low-risk mothers.

[2] Albert D. Haverkamp, M.D., "The Evaluation of Continuous Fetal Heart Rate and Monitoring in High-risk Pregnancy," *American Journal of Obstetrics and Gynecology* 125:3, 310–17 (June 1976). In addition to the findings reported in the text of this chapter, Haverkamp felt that the use of monitors did indeed add to the Cesarean rate of the women included in his study.

Ian M. Kelso, et al., "An Assessment of Continuous Fetal Heart Monitoring in Labor," *American Journal of Obstetrics and Gynecology* 131(5): 526–32 (July 1, 1978). This study also showed an increase in Cesareans among the women who were monitored by electronic fetal monitors, but Kelso felt that this could not be directly attributed to the monitors alone.

How does an individual doctor respond if fetal distress is detected by an electronic monitor? Most accept this as an indication that something may be wrong, not an indication that an immediate Cesarean delivery will be necessary. (Of course, this depends on the severity of the distress shown.) Sometimes there are steps that can be taken to correct distress before a Cesarean is the only answer. If oxytocin is being given, dosages will often be lowered or stopped altogether. It has been shown that lying on your back can cause a drop in blood pressure, which lowers the supply of oxygen to your baby, resulting in distress. You may be asked to move around for a time in an attempt to bring your blood pressure back to normal. Epidural anesthesia may cause a drop in your blood pressure also, and anesthetic may be discontinued. At times, you may be given a drug to relax your uterus.

Now many doctors take a tiny blood sample from your baby's scalp to check the levels of oxygen as well as the pH in your infant's blood, since many times a drop in fetal heart rate on an electronic monitor does not mean that distress is actually occurring. In fact, the NICHHD Task Force referred to above concluded: "EFM should be regarded not as a diagnostic test but as a screening test because of the large number of false-positive findings." (False-positive means cases where distress as shown by the monitor turned out to be inaccurate.)

Are electronic fetal monitors adding to the Cesarean birthrate? It is really difficult to assess the impact EFMs have had on the rising Cesarean rate, since their introduction coincided with other changes in obstetrical care, such as the practice of delivering almost all first breech babies abdominally. It would be a mistake to say that the monitors themselves cause Cesareans. Inappropriate interpretation of the machine's findings, however, is certainly the reason some Cesareans are done.

Some couples are so concerned about the use of monitors and the rising Cesarean rate that they would like their doctor to agree categorically not to use either type of electronic monitor for the birth. This position is probably unreasonable and perhaps even dangerous. Indeed, there are women who have had a perfectly normal pregnancy, who begin labor very routinely, yet run into problems before the baby can be vaginally delivered. There are other ways of evaluating a baby during labor, however, than by the routine use of EFMs. It is the routine use of these monitors that should be questioned, not their benefits when specific problems arise.

Many women object to the routine use of monitors during labor because they "invade" the body at an extremely sensitive time. Once the monitor is attached, they feel that their labor is controlled by the machine.

> It was such a strange feeling to be sharing a room with a blinking, beeping machine. I asked the doctor if anyone ever died of electrocution before the baby was delivered, but he didn't laugh. Each time the sound from the monitor changed, everyone became riveted to the machine. I felt like Alice in Wonderland. I was shrinking and the monitor was growing larger.

It is within the realm of our technology to design an effective monitor that does not include wires running from machine to mother. Any benefits of continuous monitoring could be preserved, and the problems of limited movement, wires, and interference would be eliminated. Prototypes of such monitors have been developed. In fact, this principle was used to monitor the hearts of astronauts while in space. Currently such monitors are prohibitively expensive, but their development is possible. The same people who design this equipment rarely must use it while in labor. Perhaps once more empathy develops for consumer objections to the machines now available, more economical means of production will be found.

# FETAL BLOOD-GAS DETERMINATIONS

### What Happens
Your doctor will insert a small cone-shaped instrument (much like the insertion of a speculum during a Pap smear) into your vagina and gently remove a few drops of blood from your baby's scalp.

*Why*

This test is used most frequently to confirm or deny distress patterns detected during internal monitoring. The baby's blood can be tested for amounts of oxygen, carbon dioxide, and pH levels. pH measures the acidity and alkalinity of the blood. If the pH level is too low, it indicates that distress is indeed occurring.

*Considerations*

You may feel slight discomfort while the blood sample is being taken, especially if it is done during a contraction. Relaxation techniques taught in childbirth classes are helpful.

This test is increasingly being used to avert unnecessary Cesarean deliveries. If the blood sample does not confirm distress, your doctor has time to attempt to correct whatever problems are occurring. When blood-gas determinations show that your baby is in severe distress, they support the decision for Cesarean birth.

Rare complications include infections at the site where the blood was drawn, and bleeding from your baby's scalp.

# X RAY PELVIMETRY

*What Happens*

Usually this test is done after you have been in labor for a time, although it sometimes is used late in pregnancy. You will be taken to a room in the X ray department of the hospital. Two views are usually taken, one front view to measure the transverse (east–west) diameters of your pelvis, and one side view to measure the longitudinal (north–south) diameters. If you are in labor, the views are taken during a contraction while you hold your breath.

*Why*

X ray pelvimetry is often used if cephalo-pelvic disproportion is suspected. It can measure your pelvis and the approximate size of your baby's head, as well as indicate the position of your baby's head in your uterus. By studying the films, your doctor can also gain a better understanding of the overall structure of your pelvis.

### Considerations

It seemed as if I had been in labor forever. I was definitely losing my sense of humor. My doctor was beginning to look grave and my husband looked exhausted. The doctor said he was sending us down to X ray to have some pictures taken. I was sort of happy that someone was finally doing something. I was scared too, though. Somehow leaving that labor room seemed like deserting the only familiar place we had.

When this test occurs after many hours of labor it can cause anxiety for both parents. Moving to another room may disturb your concentration if you are using prepared childbirth techniques. It may also make you feel insecure for a time. Checking the size of your pelvis certainly does not mean a Cesarean will occur. Your doctor wants to establish as accurately as possible why your labor is not progressing, and this is one tool available.

The radiation received from X ray pelvimetry is very limited, and the value often outweighs the risks for you and your baby.

## ULTRASOUND OR SONOGRAPHY

### What Happens

Ultrasound is usually done on an outpatient basis during your pregnancy, but sometimes is used after you have labored for a time. If it is done early in your pregnancy you will be asked to arrive at the hospital with a full bladder or drink a large quantity of water immediately before the procedure. This is so your bladder can serve as a reference point for the technician. The room where the test is given may be relatively dark so the technician can more easily view the ultrasound screen. Your abdomen will be swabbed with mineral oil, which increases the conductivity of the sound waves. You will lie flat on a table, and an instrument that looks like a microphone will be gently rubbed back and forth over your abdomen. Sound waves far above the range of human hearing are beamed toward your uterus. When the sound waves encounter either your baby or the placenta, they bounce back, and the echoes are recorded as an echogram on a screen called an oscilloscope. If a permanent record is desired, a Polaroid camera will be used. (It is often possible to obtain one of these records. Although it is not a picture in the usual sense, it is exciting to see the outline of your baby.) The test is quiet and painless, although you may feel stiff after a time. Feel free to request a break, and do some stretching to relieve the strain of lying still. Usually the person conducting the test explains each step as you go along. If this doesn't happen, feel free to ask any questions that occur to you.

## Why

Ultrasound can provide an image of your baby and your placenta. This gives the doctor needed information about the size of your baby in relation to the amount of time spent in the uterus. (You may hear your doctor refer to "gestational age.") Your doctor may use this information as one means to judge when a repeat Cesarean should be scheduled. Ultrasound can be used to detect multiple births, abnormal positions, and as an aid in confirming suspected cephalo-pelvic disproportion. This test is frequently used prior to amniocentesis to establish the position of your baby and placenta before the needle is inserted and amniotic fluid is withdrawn. (See following discussion.)

## Considerations

Ultrasound is seldom used by itself to determine your due date, since it is accurate within only two weeks either before or after the time your baby is actually due. Ultrasound does not entail radiation, as do X rays, which were previously the only means of determining the size or position of a baby during pregnancy. The amount of radiation a baby was exposed to was minimal, but since most doctors prefer to avoid all exposure if possible, many now use ultrasound when it is available. Recently, the Food and

Drug Administration has issued a "Draft Notice of Intent to Propose Rules and Develop Recommendations Related to Diagnostic Ultrasound Equipment." The agency currently warns against the use of pregnant women during demonstrations of the equipment. There are no studies at present that prove that ultrasound is unsafe. However, there will be ongoing tests, and current periodicals will be good sources of up-to-date findings.

## AMNIOCENTESIS

### *What Happens*

This test can be performed either on an outpatient basis at your hospital or in your doctor's office. If done immediately after ultrasound, as it usually is, the mineral oil will be washed off your abdomen and it will be swabbed with a small amount of antiseptic solution, which reduces surface bacteria. Towels will be draped over your abdomen to keep the area sterile. Usually a small amount of anesthetic is injected near the place where the fluid is to be withdrawn. After this has taken effect, a very thin, long needle is inserted through your abdomen into your uterus. A syringe is attached, and fluid is pulled up into the needle. The needle is then withdrawn and a small Band-Aid may be placed over the area. The amniotic fluid that has been collected is sent to a laboratory to be tested. Results can take a few hours, days, or even weeks, depending on the location of the lab and the test or tests to be done.

### *Why*

Your baby is continuously shedding cells and other substances into the amniotic fluid that surrounds him. Amniocentesis provides amniotic fluid that can be tested to reveal a great deal about your baby. If amniocentesis is done about the fourth month of your pregnancy, it can give you and your doctor information about the presence of such serious birth defects as mongolism (Down's Syndrome), Tay-Sachs Disease and Spina Bifida. This test can also be used to determine the sex of the baby although it is seldom performed solely for this purpose.

When amniocentesis is used late in pregnancy it is usually as an aid to verify your due date before a Cesarean delivery. Your doctor is seeking information about the maturity of your infant, especially the lungs. Mature lungs do not necessarily mean your baby will not be premature; it does mean that he will have a much better chance for survival should delivery be performed, since almost certainly he will not have RDS (respiratory distress syndrome). RDS, or hyaline membrane disease, is an extremely serious illness that occurs primarily in premature babies. A recent study of one hundred cases of RDS found that nine of them were associated with Cesarean deliveries that were done without maturity studies.[3]

One important test that can be done on the amniotic fluid to measure the maturity of your baby's lungs is a determination of the lecithin (L)/sphingomyelin (S) ratio. These are lipids (fatty substances) contained in surfactant, a chemical substance that is synthesized by the cells of the lungs and secreted into the amniotic fluid. Once surfactant is present in sufficient amounts, the small air sacs that make up your baby's lungs can more easily remain expanded, allowing him to exchange oxygen and carbon dioxide on his own. Until approximately the thirty-fifth week of your pregnancy, these two substances appear in equal amounts. After this time, the amount of lecithin increases until it reaches ratios ranging from two to one to four to one. With very few exceptions, an L/S of two (or more) to one means that the baby will be able to breathe on his own without problems.

Because there are exceptions (notably babies of diabetic

[3] Robert Goldenberg and Kathleen Nelson, "Iatrogenic Respiratory Distress Syndrome," *American Journal of Obstetrics and Gynecology* 6:611 (Nov. 15, 1975). This retrospective study of one hundred cases of respiratory distress syndrome determined that unwarranted or untimely physician intervention in the pregnancy was responsible for fifteen of the cases and was possibly responsible for an additional eighteen cases. The fifteen cases involving unwarranted intervention included nine scheduled Cesareans that were done without maturity studies.

mothers), more specific analyses of surfactant are being performed in some labs. These involve the determination of various components of lecithin. Currently this test is available only in research labs and perinatal centers.

The shake or "foam" test, a simpler measure of pulmonary surfactant, is a less specific way to measure the L/S and as such is not as frequently used.

### Considerations

Many doctors encourage women who are having repeat Cesareans to wait for labor to begin spontaneously rather than schedule delivery. However, if the birth is scheduled, it is essential that some means be used to determine the baby's maturity because sometimes a scheduled Cesarean is done before the baby is ready. Although there are a variety of ways to try to determine the maturity of your infant, most of them are not entirely accurate. The date of conception can be inaccurate, even if you and your doctor have the best of intentions. The date of quickening (the first time you feel movement) and the first hearing of a heartbeat include too many variables to insure delivery of a mature infant. Even X rays and ultrasound provide only general estimates of your baby's maturity and must be used with other procedures to be accurate. At this time, establishing the L/S is the most reliable way to predict how your baby's lungs will function if delivered.

Although the routine use of amniocentesis is debatable, the risks associated with it are in some measure counterbalanced by the risk of needless premature birth.

There are alternatives to amniocentesis. One, of course, is to permit women who are to have repeat Cesarean deliveries to go into labor. Some obstetricians do allow this, especially if you live relatively close to the hospital. The use of amniocentesis will be reduced, too, as more women deliver vaginally rather than by repeat Cesareans.

Amniocentesis can be an emotionally trying experience for the mother. The equipment used is rather intimidating, and it is difficult to think about a long needle being inserted into the abdomen, although it is very safe when performed by a knowledgeable

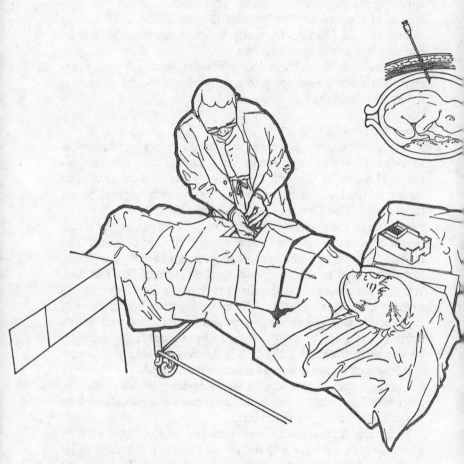

During amniocentesis the doctor withdraws a small amount of amniotic fluid. Tests of the fluid can reveal valuable information about your baby.

individual. Most women find it is not painful, but many experience feelings of pressure and some feel discomfort as the needle is inserted. It might be helpful to have your husband or a friend with you during the procedure. Check beforehand to clear this with your doctor or hospital. You will probably find that the anticipation is worse than the procedure itself, especially if you have practiced relaxation techniques beforehand.

Many women are worried that their baby might be poked with the needle used to extract the fluid. If the baby receives a slight poke there is usually no problem, unless it occurs in a vital area. The skill of the obstetrician in establishing the baby's position as well as the use of ultrasound have made such occurrences extremely rare. There is a slight chance of infection from the procedure as well as minimal risk that labor may begin following amniocentesis. If this happens, it is usually very close to the due date. It is extremely rare that labor is precipitated by amniocentesis, and the risk of a Cesarean done without maturity studies probably outweighs the danger of beginning labor.

# FETAL ACTIVITY DETERMINATION

### What Happens
You will be asked to come to the hospital for a few hours. An external monitor will be strapped across your abdomen. Each time your baby moves, you will be asked to push a button. The monitor graphs how your baby's heart reacts during activity.

### Why
There normally is an acceleration of the baby's heartbeat as she moves. This test is done to make sure your baby's heart is reacting as it should.

### Considerations
This is a painless procedure for both mother and baby.

# NONSTRESS TEST

*What Happens*
This test is usually done late in your pregnancy. You will be asked to come to the hospital, and an external monitor will be strapped to your abdomen. While you are lying still, your baby's heartbeat will be graphed for twenty minutes to an hour.

*Why*
This test provides a general picture of how your pregnancy is progressing. Your doctor is especially interested in how your baby's heart reacts to spontaneous uterine contractions (you may hear them referred to as Braxton-Hicks contractions), which occur late in your pregnancy. If any abnormalities appear during this time, there may be a need for further testing.

*Considerations*
This test is also a painless procedure for mother and baby.

# OXYTOCIN CHALLENGE TEST OR STRESS TEST (OCT)

*What Happens*
When you have a stress test you come to the hospital for a few hours. Again an external monitor is used, but this time an intravenous (IV) infusion will be started, and enough oxytocin (a synthetic hormone) will be added to the drip to produce three good contractions during a ten-minute period. Your baby's heart rate will be monitored during these contractions.

*Why*
A stress test is often used if your doctor is concerned about how the placenta is functioning. This is likely to happen if you have diabetes, kidney disease, high blood pressure, or if your baby is

more than two weeks past due. Your doctor may also order this test if there have been abnormalities during a nonstress test or if he or she has reason to be concerned about how your baby's heart would withstand the stress of labor.

If your baby's heart rate pattern in response to the contractions is normal, your pregnancy will probably continue for a while longer, usually from five to seven days, at which time the test will be repeated. If signs of fetal distress occur during this test, they indicate that your baby may be in jeopardy, and further testing may be done, or your Cesarean will be scheduled.

### Considerations
Stress tests usually will not be advised for a woman with a history of premature labor. There are rare instances when this amount of oxytocin initiates true labor. The test is not painful, but it does produce discernible contractions, much like Braxton-Hicks contractions. Breathing techniques used in prepared childbirth will help you relax during the test.

## ESTRIOL LEVELS

### What Happens
Estriol levels may be checked by testing either your blood or your urine. If blood tests are used, you will come to your doctor's office so a small amount of blood can be drawn. If urine estriols are to be checked, you will be asked to collect your total urinary output for twenty-four hours and bring it to your doctor's office or the hospital lab for testing. This must be repeated anywhere from every two to three days to a week to ten days, since estriol levels can vary widely within a short time span.

### Why
Estriol is a hormone jointly produced by the mother, the baby, and the placenta. It passes through the placenta into the mother's bloodstream and ultimately is excreted through the kidneys. Nor-

mally, as pregnancy continues, the level of estriol in the mother's system increases. A drop in estriol levels may signal problems and indicates a need for further testing, or delivery of the baby in the near future. Estriol levels may be monitored in women with diabetes or hypertension. Estriols may also be checked if a woman's pregnancy has gone beyond her due date.

### Considerations

It is important to collect every bit of urine during the twenty-four hours of the test period. If you do forget a specimen, tell the doctor so that this can be taken into account. One or two missed specimens can drastically alter the results of the test.

> I don't know why collecting urine bothered me but it sure did. Maybe it just seemed like the final indignity. I understood why the doctor wanted me to do it. I was even glad that there was a way to check how things were going for this baby I wanted so badly. But I sure didn't like doing it.

There is general agreement that checking estriol levels is a valuable tool in certain pregnancies. Nonetheless, it can be inconvenient to store a full day's output of urine in a gallon jug in your refrigerator, especially toward the end of your pregnancy, when urination seems to be one of your major occupations. It can be tiring to drive to your doctor's office or the laboratory early in the morning when your energy is low and time is precious to you. Repeated estriol checks can also be expensive, and many medical insurance plans do not cover all the costs involved. The inconvenience and expense must be weighed against the necessary information that can only be had from this particular test.

## INDUCTION OF LABOR

### What Happens

You will be asked to admit yourself to the hospital, and routine preparations for birth will be performed. (See Chapter Five for a complete discussion.) An IV will be started and an oxytocic drug will be added to the solution or "drip." Medical personnel often call this a "Pit drip," referring to Pitocin, an oxytocic drug commonly used for inductions.

## Why

There are some sound medical reasons to attempt an induction of labor. Women who have diabetes, kidney disease, hypertension, toxemia, and certain other problems may benefit when their pregnancy is ended shortly before their estimated due date. Pregnancies that continue beyond forty-two weeks may also need this medical intervention for the baby's well-being.

## Considerations

Inducing labor is one way of bringing about early delivery, and properly used it can be a useful, life-saving tool. An induction is more likely to be successful under some circumstances than others. You should have had regular menstrual cycles and be as certain as humanly possible of the date of conception. Your due date should ideally be very close, and your cervix should be partially dilated and thinned out. Your baby's head should be engaged in your pelvis and your baby should be of good size. There are times when other medical indications, such as diabetes, will warrant induction, even though some of the above criteria cannot be met. When this happens, the induction may not stimulate productive labor and a Cesarean may be necessary. In these cases, however, it is usually much safer for the baby to be delivered by Cesarean than to remain in the uterus.

Recent labeling of oxytocic drugs was designed to eliminate any but medically indicated inductions. The label states: "[The specific drug] is indicated for the medical rather than the elective induction of labor. Available data and information are inadequate to determine the benefits to risks considerations in the use of the drug product for elective inductions." Elective induction of labor is defined as "the initiation of labor for convenience in an individual with a term pregnancy who is free of medical indications." The new requirements also state that the drug must be given intravenously. Pills that dissolve in the mouth have now been banned. An automatic infusion pump or similar device must be used and the mother must be closely watched by trained personnel who frequently monitor the strength of contractions and the infant's heart.

# FOUR

# Anesthesia

Few would argue about the place of anesthesia in Cesarean delivery. The surgical nature of the birth compels you to accept it as part of your birth experience. Although there are a few times when acupuncture, hypnosis, or local anesthetics are used, most women receive either regional or general anesthesia for a Cesarean delivery. Regional (sometimes called conduction) anesthesia as it is used for Cesareans numbs you from the chest down so you are awake during the birth. There are two types of regional anesthesia, spinal and epidural. General anesthesia causes total unconsciousness, so you see, feel, and hear nothing while your baby is being delivered.

Parents often have questions and fears about anesthesia. Many parents are concerned about what kind of anesthesia they will have because it has such an effect on their birth experience. Will you have regional or general anesthesia? The decision is usually based on three considerations: the medical condition of mother and baby; the preferences and policies of doctors and hospital; and your preferences.

## YOUR CONDITION—YOUR BABY'S CONDITION

Sometimes the reason you are having a Cesarean delivery also determines the type of anesthesia you will be given. In many instances, general anesthesia will be used—either because it is considered safer in the light of the medical conditions present, or because it is faster to administer.

One of the risks associated with regional anesthesia is lowered maternal blood pressure. Since vaginal bleeding also causes a drop in blood pressure, women who have had or are having bleeding are thought to be much safer when general anesthesia is used. If you have high blood pressure, toxemia or pre-eclampsia, general anesthesia may be considered preferable also. Women with a history of back trouble or spinal or nervous system diseases may not be considered safe candidates for regional anesthesia. More rarely, a rash on or near the area where regional anesthetic would be injected prohibits use of this type of anesthesia.

Your baby's medical condition can also be the determining factor in the choice of anesthesia. Sometimes it is necessary to deliver a baby very quickly. General anesthesia is much faster to administer than a regional. General anesthesia becomes effective almost immediately, while a spinal can take three to six minutes and an epidural up to twenty minutes to numb a woman sufficiently so the surgery can begin. If your baby is in severe distress, your doctor may feel that it is not safe to wait that long to deliver the baby.

## PROFESSIONAL PREFERENCES AND POLICIES
(*Obstetricians, Anesthesiologists,*[1] *and Hospitals*)

Although regional anesthesia is being used more for Cesarean deliveries than ever before, general anesthesia is still given to about half of the women who have surgical deliveries. Since anesthesia used for Cesarean delivery affects two people, mother and baby,

---

[1] For our purposes, the word "anesthesiologist" is used to designate either the nurse anesthetist (a nurse trained in the use of anesthesia) or anesthesiologist (a doctor who specializes in anesthesia).

doctors weigh the risks and benefits to both as they make their decision.

There are doctors who have serious reservations about the use of regional anesthesia for any Cesarean delivery. They are particularly concerned about the risk of hypotension (lowered blood pressure) in the mother. Those who disagree feel that this problem, while not to be ignored, is minimal and can be controlled through proper administration of the anesthetic and careful monitoring of the mother during delivery. Doctors who support the use of regional anesthesia often point out that there is a risk of aspiration (ingesting fluid into the lungs) or cardiovascular complications that can occur when general anesthesia is used.

There is concern over the effects of general anesthesia on the baby. An infant born under general anesthesia may be sleepier than one not exposed to these agents. Newer techniques have reduced the number of times this happens, however, and if it does occur it usually passes fairly quickly.

Actually the risks involved in either type of anesthesia are extremely small when used by competent medical professionals. However, an increasing number of doctors are becoming more sensitive to the fact that it is important to many women that they be awake for the birth of their baby. Regional anesthesia is now chosen by many doctors because of its benefits for the entire Cesarean family.

There are times when, though your obstetrician would support the use of regional anesthesia, other factors will stand in the way. Your doctor may be limited by the policy of the anesthesia department at the hospital where you deliver, since some units do all Cesarean deliveries under general anesthesia. In hospitals that provide both types of anesthesia, the final decision rests with the anesthesiologist. In these cases, the preference and competence of the anesthesiologist who attends your birth will be the deciding factors. Not all anesthesiologists are trained to give regional anesthetics. Your choice may be limited unless your hospital has twenty-four hour coverage by anesthesiologists experienced in obstetrical anesthetics. If the anesthesiologist refuses you a spinal because he or she has not been trained in that type of anesthesia, you have no alternative but to be guided by his or her judgment.

## THE PARENTS' REASONS

Assuming that you and your baby would be in no particular danger from the use of one anesthesia or the other, and assuming that both your obstetrician and the anesthesiologist are willing to use either type, your choice will be the determining factor. If you have the chance to exercise this choice, much of your decision will probably revolve around a desire to be awake for the birth of your baby or a wish to be asleep until delivery is completed.

> When we learned that our second child was on the way, we decided that more than anything else we wanted to be together for the birth. My husband and I immediately began planning with our doctor. We agreed that if everything went as expected, I would have a spinal and my husband would be with me. After many months of waiting and wondering, the day finally arrived. My husband had to wait until they gave me the spinal, but then there he was, smiling and holding my hand. We talked during the delivery and we first saw our baby together.

Women who choose regional anesthesia usually do so because they wish to participate as fully as possible in the birth of their child. Since a spinal or an epidural allows a woman to be conscious during the delivery and in the recovery room, she has her own "history" of the events surrounding her baby's birth. Most hospitals that allow fathers to be present for Cesarean deliveries stipulate that the mother must be awake for the birth. Since many couples would prefer to be together for the delivery, they obviously would choose regional anesthesia.

Some women are very leery about Cesarean delivery. They may be afraid that if they are awake during the birth they will see or hear things that they wouldn't be able to cope with. They may be afraid of experiencing a great deal of pain if they don't remain unconscious through the birth. Not too many years ago, women used to request "gas" during vaginal deliveries for many of the same reasons. As more couples prepare for childbirth, fewer feel this anxious about delivery. Of course, there are major differences between vaginal birth and Cesarean delivery, but for both, the more you know about what is involved, the less frightening it becomes. Better information in traditional childbirth courses, classes for Cesarean couples, and easier access to literature about surgical delivery have done much to alleviate the "fear of the unknown" with regard to Cesarean birth.

If you think you prefer a general, learn all you can about Cesarean delivery, especially about the different kinds of anesthesia used. It is important to know as much as possible about anesthesia, for just understanding can do wonders.

## HOW YOU EXERCISE YOUR CHOICE

Even though anesthesia is so central to your birth experience, it is sometimes very difficult for parents to have much control over how the decision is made to use one type or the other. When there is a conflict between parents' wishes and professional opinion, it is usually because you want a regional form of anesthesia but you are in a hospital where general anesthesia is used as a matter of course.

Probably the best place to begin is with your own obstetrician. Discuss anesthesia thoroughly early in your pregnancy. If you find that you and your doctor have opposite views on the benefits of a particular type of anesthesia, you will have to decide whether to remain with that doctor and attempt to reach a compromise that is satisfactory to both of you, or whether you should seek other medical care.

If you are contending with a uniform anesthesia policy covering an entire hospital, it will take much energy and a lot of time to bring changes about. You may have the most success working with a group of parents concerned with family-centered Cesarean care. (Chapter Fifteen discusses how such groups are formed and operate.)

When you have an unexpected Cesarean delivery, you meet the anesthesiologist only a short time before your baby is born. You will only have time for a brief description of what is involved in anesthesia, not a lengthy discussion of the pros and cons of regional or general anesthesia.

> I know that our Lamaze instructor talked about anesthesia as well as other medication during the classes we took. I was so sure that we would have a "natural" childbirth that I just didn't really listen. Even learning about anesthesia seemed against everything my husband and I wanted for this birth. When they said that I would have a Cesarean and wanted to talk about anesthesia, I panicked. Everything I had half heard or half read came rushing back to me. I couldn't listen to the doctor and I couldn't remember enough on my own to make any decision.

It is important that you let your doctor and the hospital know how you feel about anesthesia. Even if there is not enough time to change policy before your delivery, you will help parents who have Cesarean births in the future.

## IF YOU HAVE GENERAL ANESTHESIA

General anesthesia is most often given by a combination of gases you breathe through a mask or tube and medication injected into your IV. After these have taken effect, you will be asleep and unconscious through the entire delivery.

Prior to administration of general anesthesia, you will be given oxygen through a mask. This can be a difficult moment, since the mask often smells rubbery or medicinal and it can be disconcerting to have your mouth and nose covered. Although many women think they will feel sleepy as soon as the mask is put on, this is not the case. The oxygen is given to increase the levels circulating in your blood and consequently to your baby. If you relax and breathe as normally as possible, it can be given very quickly. Next, an injection of a barbiturate is put into your IV and you will be completely asleep within fifteen to twenty seconds. You are not actually unconscious at this point. You are simply asleep, making it easier for the anesthetic to be administered. A second injection, containing a muscle relaxant, will be placed into the IV. This drug relaxes your entire body and causes temporary paralysis. The use of muscle relaxants reduces the amount of anesthetic and narcotics needed for the delivery. (These relaxants do not cross the placenta in large enough amounts to affect your baby.)

At this time a rubber tube is inserted into your throat. Since you are temporarily paralyzed, the anesthesiologist can manage your breathing for you through the tube. Next you will be given a mixture of oxygen and nitrous oxide, either through the tube or through the mask used to give you oxygen earlier. The gases are inhaled into your lungs and absorbed into your circulating blood. As the blood circulates through your body to your brain in sufficient amounts, it causes total unconsciousness.

### Considerations if You Have General Anesthesia
One of the most serious risks to the mother from general anesthesia is that she might vomit and aspirate (ingest) liquid into the lungs. If surgery is planned, as in the case of a repeat Cesarean delivery, the mother is instructed not to eat anything for eight to twelve hours before delivery. If you have an unexpected Cesarean, this cannot be as easily controlled. Even if you have not eaten for many hours prior to delivery, it is possible for some food to be left in your stomach. The tube (called an endotracheal tube, since it passes through your larynx and into the trachea, which leads directly to the lungs) now used with general anesthesia eliminates much of this risk, since the entrance to the lungs is blocked and any fluid can be suctioned by the anesthesiologist. If you become partially conscious while the tube is still in place you may experi-

ence some coughing or vomiting. Also, after it is removed, you may have a sore throat for a few days.

You will experience a certain amount of confusion as you wake up from general anesthesia. You may come into and out of consciousness and later find it difficult to reconstruct what happened immediately following your baby's birth. Often it seems that you have slept only a few minutes when the nurse once again comes to check your progress.

It may be difficult to connect with your mate for a few hours following the delivery. This feeling of general grogginess can continue for a few hours or even a few days, especially while you are taking medication for pain. Some women experience strange dreams or hallucinations while "coming out of" general anesthesia. Often this can cause feelings of uncertainty about what has happened, and in a few cases women are very panicky. Any time general anesthesia is used it is extremely helpful to have a supportive person with you during your stay in the recovery room and your transfer to the postpartum floor.

I was so glad Joe was with me for the time in recovery. I wanted to sleep more than anything in the whole world but I kept waking up when the nurse came by. It was good to see him there and have him hold my hand. Later, he could tell me about the baby and the nurses and how happy our doctor was to have delivered her.

There is still some concern about the effects of general anesthesia on the baby. Until fairly recently, a baby born under general anesthesia was sleepier than those born while regional anesthesia was used. A baby is less apt to be sleepy with techniques recently developed for general anesthesia. When a baby is sleepy, the grogginess usually disappears within a short time, unless there are other problems occurring at the same time. A baby born under general anesthesia may also have more difficulty nursing for the first few hours, since general anesthesia may repress a baby's sucking instinct. You certainly can nurse your baby, but you may just have to be patient while her appetite improves.

## IF YOU HAVE SPINAL ANESTHESIA

Spinal anesthesia is a regional or conduction anesthesia that numbs you from the chest down. Spinal anesthesia temporarily paralyzes you in this same area.

You will probably be asked to curl up on your side on the operating table. You will be asked to pull your knees up toward your chest and keep your back rounded. As an alternative, some doctors ask you to sit up and bend down as far as you are able. It may be difficult to imagine yourself in either position at this point in your pregnancy, but a nurse will be there to help you.

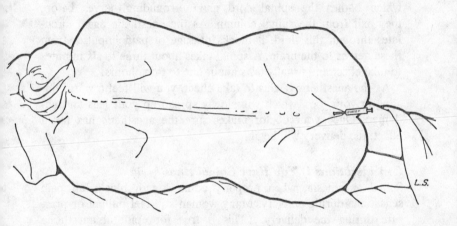

*Administration of Regional Anesthesia* The mother is lying on her side with her knees curled up (a nurse will help you hold this position). The anesthesiologist injects the anesthesia into her lower back.

They told me I had to lie on my side to have the spinal. I really didn't want to move anywhere and felt as if this were the final straw. It seemed like only minutes after the injection that my legs were getting numb. When the feeling reached my abdomen, it was the greatest relief I have ever felt in my life. I finally believed I could make it through this delivery.

Your back will be washed with a sterile solution, usually very cold, and it will be draped with sterile cloths. Next, you will be given an injection of a small amount of local anesthetic (such as Novocain) to numb the area where the spinal will be given. Once this takes effect, you will receive a very small dose of the anesthetic to check for allergic reaction and placement of the needle. The anesthesiologist will then give the full dose of medication, using a very narrow needle for the injection. The needle penetrates the dura and the arachnoid tissue layers that completely surround your spinal cord. This space contains cerebrospinal fluid, which bathes the spinal cord and surrounding nerves before they exit from the spinal column. As the anesthetic agent circulates through this fluid, it blocks passage of pain impulses from these nerves to the brain. A spinal takes about three to six minutes to take effect and usually lasts about one to three hours.

As the anesthetic begins to take effect, you will feel a warm tingling in your toes, which will slowly spread up your legs and abdomen. Once your doctor makes sure the anesthetic has taken effect, the delivery will begin.

### Considerations if You Have Spinal Anesthesia

Spinal anesthesia, when properly administered, blocks all pain sensations during delivery. Many women still feel pulling or pressure during the delivery. (This is true for epidural anesthesia also.) If they are unprepared for this possibility they may be concerned that the anesthetic is not working properly. However, many women who knew what to expect report that feeling their baby being born was absolutely terrific! The momentary discomfort was negligible compared to the joy of knowing their baby was really arriving.

During our childbirth classes, the instructor had talked about feeling something with spinals. It made me uneasy at the time, since I thought anesthesia meant you wouldn't feel a thing. When the time came, it was great. I let out a whoop of real joy. Here was my baby and I felt him coming out.

Of the two regional anesthesias used for Cesarean delivery—spinals and epidurals—spinal anesthetic is easier to administer. However, there is a higher incidence of side effects connected with its use.

The side effect that happens most frequently is a drop in the mother's blood pressure (hypotension). This occurs because the muscles and blood vessels in the anesthetized area of the body relax, allowing the blood to pool rather than return to the heart. Many times the operating table is tilted very slightly or the woman's hip is elevated a bit to aid circulation and prevent hypotension. Sometimes extra fluids are given by IV before the spinal is administered in order to increase the volume of fluid circulating in the mother's body. If the drop in blood pressure is severe, mild stimulants can be used to contract the blood vessels.

Since your intercostal muscles (the muscles between the ribs) are frequently affected by a spinal, your breathing may seem shallow or labored to you. Sometimes, if you move or cough while the injection is being given, the anesthetic can be forced higher than necessary in your spinal column. There is always a nurse to assist you while you are being given the anesthetic. She will help you remain still and remind you not to push during the injection. Once the spinal has taken effect, if you feel you are having trouble breathing, tell the anesthesiologist. Although you may be feeling very uncomfortable, the fact is that if you can talk, you can breathe.

The side effect of spinal anesthesia that most women are aware of is the infamous spinal headache. The headache can happen if a small amount of spinal fluid leaks through the hole made by the injection. This results in a shortage of fluid in the spinal column so that your brain presses on the bottom of your skull while you are standing. Spinal headaches occur very infrequently now that a very thin needle is used to give the anesthetic. Currently, about 1 to 2 per cent of women who are delivered under spinal anesthesia have this complication. Usually it persists for one to two days, al-

though it can last longer. If you do have a spinal headache, steps
will be taken to alleviate your discomfort. Often extra fluids are
given to build up the supply you have lost. Pain medication and
bed rest will be advised until the headache subsides. The practice
of keeping women flat on their backs for eight to twenty-four
hours after surgery as a way of avoiding spinal headaches has
been eliminated by many hospitals. Lying flat does not seem to
prevent a headache from happening, but can offer relief if one
does occur.

In addition to side effects, there are a few other aspects of spinal anesthesia with which you should be familiar. Some doctors
routinely give a sleeping medication or sedative once the delivery
is completed and suturing has begun. They may feel that since the
repair takes much longer (twenty to forty-five minutes) than the
birth (three to ten minutes) and the "main event" is over, it
would be best for you to sleep during this time. Many women
prefer that such medication not be given. They want to be alert
not only in the operating room but also during their time in the
recovery area so they can enjoy their first moments of parenthood.

It is estimated that spinals are effective about 95 per cent of the
time. (This is known as the "take rate.") If your spinal is not
fully effective and there is enough time, you may be given a second dose of the spinal. Another alternative is to use local anesthetics for the delivery, and then some type of general anesthesia
is given while suturing is done. Some doctors immediately administer general anesthesia if a spinal is not effective.


## IF YOU HAVE EPIDURAL ANESTHESIA

Epidural anesthesia is the other type of regional or conduction
anesthesia used for Cesarean delivery. Although both epidurals
and spinals numb the lower half of your body, epidural anesthesia
allows you to move the affected areas.

Spinals and epidurals are given in much the same way. You

will be asked to curl up on your side or bend down while the anesthetic is being given. You will be prepped before your epidural and your back will be swabbed with an antiseptic solution, then draped with cloths. The needle for an epidural penetrates until just before the dura (the tough membranes that enclose the spinal column). After the needle has been correctly placed, a tiny plastic tube is threaded through and the needle itself is removed. The tubing is taped to your side or shoulder and left in place during the delivery. This makes it possible to give you additional anesthetic as needed. The anesthetic agent spreads through the epidural space to the nerves surrounding the spinal column. As levels of anesthesia increase, the nerves are blocked from sending pain impulses to the brain. An epidural takes from ten to twenty minutes to become effective and can be prolonged as needed.

### Considerations if You Have Epidural Anesthesia
More drug is needed for epidural anesthesia than for spinals. Spinals are placed in direct contact with the nerves that are to be blocked, while epidurals must slowly diffuse to those nerves. The area where the anesthetic is injected is rich in veins, and the drugs are quickly absorbed into your bloodstream. This increases the chance of some drugs reaching your baby. There are a variety of drugs commonly used for epidurals. The drugs now most often used for epidurals have little or no effect on the baby.

Some of the problems associated with spinal anesthesia can be avoided if epidurals are used. Although hypotension can occur because of an epidural, it usually happens much more slowly than when spinal anesthesia is used and therefore is easier to control. If the anesthetic begins to wear off, additional amounts can easily be given, since the tubing stays in place. The anesthesia can also be prolonged, so you can hold and nurse your baby while you are still comfortable.

There are drawbacks to the use of epidural anesthesia. The first is the "take rate" mentioned above. Since everyone's anatomy is different, it is difficult to predict just how effective an epidural will be for any particular person. Sometimes numbing is spotty, leaving the incision site with partial feeling. Because of this, about 6 to 8 per cent of women who initially receive epidurals need some further type of anesthesia.

Epidurals are more difficult to give than either spinal or general anesthesia. A highly trained anesthesiologist must be on duty for this type of anesthesia to be used. Incorrect placement of an epidural injection can cause "total spinal anesthesia," a name that may be misleading since it refers to a complication of both spinal and epidural anesthesia. "Total spinal anesthesia" happens very rarely, but when it does the woman's breathing is interfered with. Usually she is given a general anesthetic, so the anesthesiologist can manage her breathing for her until she is able to breathe once again on her own. (This condition happens even more rarely during spinal anesthesia.)

Although there is not a specific "epidural headache," an accidental dural puncture may cause a particularly severe headache. Accidental puncture (in good hands) runs in the one to two per cent area, and the risk of a headache in these cases would be high.

# FIVE

# Getting Ready for the Delivery

You may know months ahead of time that you will have a Cesarean delivery, or you may find out only days, hours, or minutes before your baby is born. Whatever your situation, there are certain preparations that must be completed before you can deliver your baby. If your Cesarean is planned, the preparations are usually done the evening before and the morning of the day your baby is scheduled to be born. You will have enough time to understand what is happening to you, as well as to prepare emotionally for surgical birth. If your Cesarean is unexpected, you may be trying to cope with your feelings about Cesarean birth as well as blood tests, catheters, and surgical release forms.

The hours leading up to my first Cesarean are a blur now. I remember a lot of people coming and going. They all seemed to want something from me: blood, my signature, or an arm for an IV to be started. When I went to the hospital for the birth of our second child, I was really more apprehensive about the things that would happen before the baby was born than the delivery itself. But I had lots of time. Everyone answered my questions and explained everything that was being done. It was a totally different experience from the first time.

Many of the things that are done to prepare you for a Cesarean delivery are done routinely before any operation. The hospital staff will probably be most matter-of-fact as they perform the various tests and procedures to prepare for your delivery. But these same routines may cause stress and confusion for Cesarean parents—especially if surgical delivery was unexpected. Even if you are having a scheduled Cesarean, you will probably have many questions. These preparations are now leading up to the birth of *your* baby, and that's much different than reading about them!

Pre-operative routines vary from hospital to hospital. The sequence in which you are readied differs, as well as the location of many of the tests (your room or a laboratory, for example). Also, not everything included in this chapter will necessarily happen before your delivery, since not all hospitals use all the tests and procedures mentioned here.

## COMING TO THE HOSPITAL

Since most planned Cesareans are scheduled for an early morning hour (7:30 A.M. or 8:00 A.M. is typical), most women are asked to check into the hospital the afternoon or evening prior to their delivery day. This way, all pre-operative procedures can be completed during this time. Some women really look forward to these hours. They find that it is restful to be away from the responsibilities of home as they await the birth of their baby.

I had been a crazy person during the last few days before my Cesarean was going to be done. I had lists for everything: food to be prepared, phone calls to make, things to be cleaned. Driving to the hospital was like crossing over a long bridge to peacefulness. I kept thinking, "If I did it, I did it. If it didn't get done, that's just too bad."

A growing number of women prefer to spend their last night before delivery in their own home, especially if they have other young children. Some doctors and hospitals will arrange for some tests to be done on an outpatient basis a day or two before the scheduled delivery. This way, the woman does not have to be admitted to the hospital until the morning her baby will be born.

We really had a good time that last night at home. John and I had wanted a second child very much, but for just those few hours we enjoyed our three person family. I knew I would be in the hospital for about a week, so I treasured that last bedtime with my daughter, too.

When you do arrive at the hospital, you will be asked to go to the admitting office to fill out a number of forms. These usually include one for general information (address, employer, etc.), insurance forms, and consent forms for surgery and anesthesia. (If you have an emergency Cesarean, you will be asked to sign these forms shortly before the birth.) The wording of the forms is rather grim to most nonmedical people. They are routinely used to formalize your consent to the surgery and inform you of any risks involved in either the operation itself or with the use of anesthesia. You may also be asked to sign a form giving your doctor permission to circumcise the baby in the event you have a boy. You will be given one or two identification bands, which will remain on your arm until after you are discharged from the hospital. Usually you are then taken to your room. In some hospitals, you will have tests done at various labs before you are brought there.

If you arrive at the hospital in labor anticipating a vaginal delivery, usually you go to the labor room while your partner visits the admitting office to fill out the necessary papers. Sometimes the time needed to park the car, walk back to the hospital, and fill out forms can seem very long. However, your mate will rejoin you as soon as he can.

## IN YOUR ROOM

If you are having a scheduled Cesarean you will have plenty of time to unpack and make yourself comfortable. It may feel strange to be one of the few women on the maternity floor still in the pregnant state. This is a good time to get your bearings. You can do some exploring and find the nursery, the shower, and other hospital "amenities" that can make your stay more comfortable. The tests that need to be done will take up only a few hours at most, so bring something from home to help pass the time.

Since you will not be allowed any food or liquid after midnight (you may hear the nurse say you are NPO—nothing by mouth), it's important that you eat a good dinner. No matter how you feel about hospital food or how nervous you feel at 5:30 P.M., eat something, or hunger may overtake you in the middle of the night.

If you are taken to a labor room in anticipation of vaginal delivery, you may find it difficult to consider it "your room." Usually you are asked to put on a hospital gown and take only those things from your suitcase you will need before your baby is born.

## TIME TO TALK TO THE STAFF

If you are having a planned Cesarean, you will probably have a visit from someone from the anesthesia department the evening before your delivery. Often this is not the same person who will attend the baby's birth, but he or she will be able to tell you what will happen when the anesthesia is given and answer any questions you have. If your Cesarean is unexpected, you will still be seen by someone from the anesthesia department soon after the decision to do a Cesarean has been made. Usually the anesthesiologist will give you a brief outline of the procedure to be used and ask that you sign an anesthesia consent form.

If you are in the hospital the afternoon before you deliver, you may be seen by your obstetrician. This is a good time to ask any last-minute questions. It is always a good idea to have a list on which you jot things down as you think of them. Countless women remember the really important question right after the doctor walks out the door.

Always feel free to ask the nurses on the floor any questions that occur to you. Even if you don't have anything specific to inquire about, the nurses can give you a good idea of "what will happen next" as you prepare for the birth of your baby.

# TESTS THAT ARE USUALLY DONE

If you are to have a planned Cesarean, the following tests will be done before your delivery, either after you are admitted to the hospital or on an outpatient basis. If you have an emergency Cesarean, some or all of these tests will be done relatively quickly once the decision to do surgery has been made.

### Blood Tests

A small amount of blood will be drawn from a vein in your arm. This will be tested for levels of blood sugar, uric acid, and hemoglobin, as well as a number of other measures of your general health. Your blood is also typed and crossmatched on the slight chance you would require a blood transfusion. (This is routine before any operation.) Although very few women need transfusions following Cesarean birth, some hospitals request that blood be donated for you prior to delivery.

### Urinalysis

You will be asked to void into a container so that your urine can be analyzed. It will be checked for infections and for protein and glucose levels. This will be done the evening or morning before an elective Cesarean. Urinalysis is routine before any delivery. You will already have provided a specimen if you expected a vaginal delivery.

### Pulmonary Function Test

You may be asked to blow into a tube to check your lung capacity. The information given by this test is especially valuable if you are to have general anesthesia. You will rarely have a pulmonary function test prior to an emergency Cesarean delivery.

### Chest X Ray

Not all hospitals require a chest X ray before a Cesarean delivery, although many still do. If an X ray is taken, it is used to check the general condition of your lungs. Again, this information is useful particularly when general anesthesia will be used. X rays are seldom done before emergency Cesareans.

## PROCEDURES AS YOU GET READY

Many of the procedures used to prepare you for delivery are the same whether you anticipate a vaginal or a Cesarean delivery.

### Temperature, Blood Pressure, and Baby's Heartbeat

Shortly after you arrive in your room, a nurse will check your temperature, blood pressure, and pulse. She will also listen for your baby's heartbeat. These procedures will be repeated often in the hours prior to your baby's birth.

> Temperature, blood pressure and pulse. Temperature, blood pressure and pulse. I was beginning to feel as though this nurse were my long-lost friend. Every time I turned around (that's really an exaggeration, but it seemed that way at the time!), she was back again to check me out. I began to wonder if they knew something I didn't.

### Shave/Prep

Some of your pubic hair will be shaved before you deliver your baby. This is done because it is impossible to remove all bacteria from hair, and the area surrounding the incision site must be kept sterile. The amount of hair that is shaved varies from hospital to hospital. Some women are shaved from the upper abdomen down to and including the pubic area. A total shave is really not necessary for a Cesarean delivery. Many women now are shaved only to a point slightly below the line where the incision will be made. It is easier to do this kind of shave and just as safe as a total shave. It is also much more comfortable for the mother when her hair begins to grow in. Many times a total shave is done only because it is routine. If you would prefer a partial shave, ask your doctor.

If you have been prepped for a vaginal delivery, your lower pubic hair will already have been shaved. When the decision is made to do a Cesarean, your abdomen will be shaved also. Sometimes women are left with only about two inches of hair across their lower abdomen, in between the two shaved areas.

### Enema

Many hospitals routinely give enemas to all women prior to birth. If you were admitted to the hospital anticipating a vaginal delivery, it will be done shortly after your arrival at the labor room. For scheduled Cesareans, it is given either the evening or morning prior to delivery.

Not all doctors and/or hospitals routinely require enemas. Some feel it is just not necessary if you have had regular bowel movements and have had nothing to eat for twelve hours prior to delivery. Others feel that it helps the mother both during surgery and during the early recovery period, when it would be uncomfortable to move the bowels. Few women look forward to an enema. It probably is not the most comfortable thing that will ever happen to you, but the idea is usually worse than the actual experience. Talk to your doctor about his or her usual practice as well as the policy of the hospital where you will deliver so at least you know what to expect.

### Catheter

A catheter is a thin tube that drains urine from your bladder. Almost all women who have Cesarean deliveries are catheterized, although the time when the catheter is inserted varies greatly from hospital to hospital. Sometimes it is put in before you leave your room or the labor room. At times it is inserted in the operating room, either before or after anesthesia. Having a catheter inserted can be mildly uncomfortable, but you shouldn't feel it once it is in place. When properly done, it takes only a few minutes for a catheter to be inserted. You will find relaxation breathing helpful during this short time.

You are catheterized so that your bladder, which usually rests right over your uterus, will remain empty and so it can easily be moved by your obstetrician during the delivery. A catheter eliminates the need for either a bedpan or trips to the bathroom in the hours immediately following the birth. It is usually removed twelve to twenty-four hours after you deliver, but in some cases it is left in place for a few days. The type of anesthesia used for delivery, your general recovery, and hospital policy determine how long you will be catheterized.

### Storing Your Personal Belongings

Shortly before you go to the operating room, a nurse will lock any jewelry, dentures, and other valuables you have with you in a safe place. If you wear glasses or contact lenses, make sure you ask to keep them with you if you are going to be awake for the delivery.

## MEDICATIONS

Even more than tests and procedures, the kinds of medication used for Cesarean birth vary from hospital to hospital and doctor to doctor. Sometimes medication is offered to women only for specific medical circumstances, and then, of course, it is beneficial. At other times certain medicines may be routinely offered to all women as they prepare to deliver. You have a responsibility not to take a medication just because it is offered to you. You have the right at any time during your hospital stay to ask why it is being given. You also have the right to refuse a specific medicine if, after understanding the reasons your doctor ordered it, you do not feel it would be of benefit to you.

## Sleeping Pills

If you are spending the night before your Cesarean in the hospital, your doctor may order a sleeping pill for you. It is entirely up to you whether you take this medication or not. Some women find a hospital a noisy place to try to get a good night's sleep. The hours from 10:00 P.M. to 7:00 A.M. can be very long if you are tense or just excited about the next day's events. Other women prefer not to use the pills, especially if they have never taken sleeping medication before. It is difficult to predict how a sleeping pill will affect you. Some women wake up rested and alert the next morning. Some feel groggy during part of the next day.

When the nurse came with the sleeping pill, I told her I didn't need it. I felt really peaceful just then and I was sure I would go right to sleep. As soon as I got into bed, all sorts of things started rushing through my mind. I suddenly remembered that I hadn't watered the plants before I left home. I wondered what I would feel like at this time tomorrow. I pictured girl babies and boy babies and tried to see if one of them looked like the baby I would deliver in the morning. About midnight I just couldn't take it anymore. I finally rang for the nurse and told her my problem. She brought the sleeping pill back and I decided it was my only alternative or I would sleep through the birth of this baby—even with spinal anesthesia!

## Sedatives

Until fairly recently, almost all Cesarean mothers were given a mild tranquilizer or sedative just before they were taken to the operating room. While these are still routinely offered in many hospitals, women who have prepared for Cesarean delivery often feel they are unnecessary. You might check with your doctor to see if he or she feels sedatives or tranquilizers are needed for any medical reasons. If this is not the case, and you would prefer not to take it, you certainly have the right to refuse this medication.

## Atropine

You may be given an injection of atropine, a drug that reduces the amount of some secretions in your body. If you are, your mouth may feel very dry and your heartbeat may speed up a bit. Atropine is not given as routinely as it once was because of concern about possible side effects.

## Antacids

Sometimes an antacid, such as Maalox, is offered shortly before birth. This is used to neutralize acid stomach contents and may help you feel better during your delivery and recovery. The antacid also reduces some of the dangers associated with aspiration, a complication of anesthesia. (See Chapter Four.)

## IV (Intravenous Infusion)

IV is hospital "shorthand" for solutions (these can be extra fluids or medications) dripped into a vein. A needle is inserted into a vein either in the back of one of your hands or in your arm. Sometimes the needle is removed and replaced with thin tubing. When the IV is being set up, the nurse may ask which hand you normally use, so it can be put in the opposite one. If she doesn't ask, feel free to tell her.

Before your delivery, you will be given fluids, usually dextrose and water, to keep you from becoming dehydrated during the surgery. These can also build up the fluid volume in your system to minimize the risk of lowered blood pressure during regional anesthesia (see discussion in Chapter Four). During your delivery the IV keeps a vein open so you can receive medication if needed. It will be used to give you Pitocin, a drug that aids uterine contractions, after your baby is born. It is difficult to predict just how long the IV will remain in place following surgery, although forty-eight to seventy-two hours is fairly standard. A lot will depend on how soon you are able to take nourishment by mouth, your general recovery, and hospital policy.

Some doctors have begun to give antibiotics routinely through the IV during Cesarean deliveries in an effort to reduce postsurgical infections and consequently the length of a mother's hospital stay. Although some recent studies suggest that infections are less frequent when antibiotics are used, many doctors question this practice. They feel that there are a number of problems involved with their routine use. There is an additional cost at the time of delivery, as well as the possibility that new types of bacteria will emerge that resist these antibiotics. There are also questions about the ability of these drugs to prevent serious postoperative infection. Doctors who oppose routine use of the antibiotics feel that other measures, such as improved sterile techniques, will be more beneficial to Cesarean women in the effort to reduce infections.

## TO YOUR DELIVERY

You are finally ready to go! Whether this Cesarean was planned or unexpected, you are now really going to have this baby. You will be taken on a rolling stretcher to the operating room, sometimes called the Cesarean birth room. There are some hospitals that allow you to walk to the operating room, if most of the preoperative procedures are not done until then. If you ride, as many women do, you may find it strange to be whisked through the halls with only a good view of the ceiling.

> I knew Bob was there beside me, but I really couldn't see him very well. Mostly I saw white ceiling tile and lights. I remember watching the IV bottle swaying as we moved along. I felt as if I were part of a procession and that there was a crowd along the side of the street watching me go by.

Most of the time your mate can go with you to the door of the surgical suite, even if he will not be present for the birth. It is great to have a familiar hand to hold as the big moment draws nearer.

# SIX

# Your Baby Is Born

It is 6:30 A.M., Monday morning. An ordinary day to most of the rest of the people in the world, but a special day to me. My new child will come into the world. Will it be a boy or a girl? Just let the baby be born a normal, healthy child.

Yesterday we made a family outing of checking Marie into the hospital. Our sons, Joshua, age five, and Jeremy, age four, waited patiently in the admitting office of Crittenton Hospital in Rochester. When they called Marie's name—through the lobby, down the corridor to X ray and lab tests, as a family we went. By making arrangements ahead of time, Marie was able to come back home with us, have Sunday dinner, and relax before actually checking into her room at eight-thirty Sunday night.

Just a few short hours ago we had our last activity as a four member family, and here I am at the hospital door to become a five member family. It's 7:00 A.M., and I check into Marie's room. The anesthesiologist talks with us both about what to expect. This being our third go-around with a Cesarean we knew some things, but are anxious to be together for this one.

Joann, a nurse from labor and delivery, comes in to be our guide through this fantastic experience. She takes me to the doctor's dressing room, where I don surgical greens. I even get a new hat and boots. Now, dressed as Ben Casey, I return to my wife's side. She is placed on a surgery cart, and off we go together.

Surgery is a cold, busy area, with half the people already asleep. Marie goes left to have her spinal. I go right to have coffee with Robert Johnson, a friend rather than my wife's doctor for the past eleven years.

Ten minutes later (it seemed longer) we are reunited in the operating room. What a surprise! This room is about fifteen foot square and I make the twelfth person in here. Marie is smiling through the mask on her face, and I get to hold her right hand. I am placed on a stool to the right side of her beautiful face, and we talk to release nervous tension. Marie can't see over the drape, but from where I sit you can see it all. But it is going so fast, and there is so much going on here. The anesthesiologist is cracking jokes, the doctors (our doctor and an assistant are both standing over my wife) are discussing who booked the OR, and Joann, our guide, is getting set up for our child.

I haven't had a chance to see what's going on with the great protrusion on my wife's stomach, and they are ready to deliver our baby. You can see them pulling and here comes a head full of black hair. By God, the baby cries! But I can't see the feet yet. There they are, and just like the rest, all pink and damp. Marie is crying and the doctors want me to tell her if it is a boy or a girl. Don't ask me those tough questions; we just had a baby and my emotions are running away with me. I can't tell. I really can't tell. The body is all swollen down there, and the cord is hanging. It's another son for our family. Our doctor quickly corrects me, and neither Mom or Dad can fully grasp the idea of a little baby girl. She is beautiful, and she is pink and she is all there. Every toe, every finger, all ears and eyes. What a pretty child! What lungs! She is still crying and so is her mother, and the squeeze of our hands together says more than any words can.

Get yourself together, Dad. Tell Marie about her all being there and being healthy and beautiful. Tell her about watching them clean her up. My God, here she comes and I can hold her. I press her cheek next to her mother's and Marie now knows what I have been smiling about for the last few minutes.

The three of us admire each other for a few minutes, and then this feminine bundle of joy wets all over her dad's new green suit. Fantastic, that part works well, too. Our little miss goes back to Joann for more preparations and a quick clean up.

You're here to watch, Dad, and look at what is going on. Everyone is smiling and they are already sewing Marie up. Where is all the blood and mess that you got yourself ready for? I never saw it, and I watched as they sewed. Marie is so thrilled with the baby, she can care less about what the doctors are doing. This is sure a lot neater than I thought it would be.

Marie is fine, the baby is fine and I am ecstatic. In the past two hours our lives have been increased in wealth and closeness beyond measure.

In a few minutes, after a great flurry of activity, your baby will be born. Many couples are now able to share Cesarean delivery—father and mother completing what they began so many months before. In hospitals where the father cannot be present for the birth, he is often able to accompany you to the door of the operating room and rejoin you in the recovery area.

Even if your mate will be present for the birth, he probably will not join you until after anesthesia has been administered and most of the other final preparations for surgery have been completed. You will have a few minutes alone while you adjust to your new surroundings. If you are to have your baby in an operating room used for general surgery, you may find you wait for a time in a pending room with a number of sleepy individuals prior to their gall bladder operation or knee surgery. Many hospitals have Cesarean birth rooms on the obstetrical floor. If this is the case in your hospital, you usually are brought directly from your room to the Cesarean birth room.

## THE CESAREAN BIRTH ROOM

There are so many things and people to take in when you are first brought into the Cesarean birth room. These areas are usually

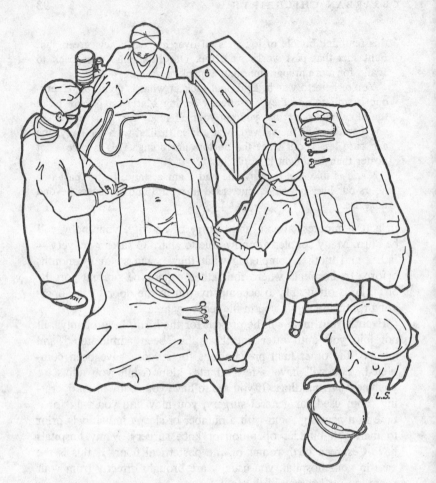

***The Cesarean Birth Room*** The medical team is in place and so
are you! The anesthesiologist is at your head. Your doctor and an
assistant are on either side. Your body is almost totally covered
with drapes except for the area where the incision will be made.
A second drape blocks your view of the incision area.

much smaller than you would have imagined, and the machines and bright lights may make you feel as if you have stumbled onto a *Star Wars* set.

There is a great deal of equipment present in any operating room, and those used for Cesarean births are certainly no exception. In fact, since the rooms are set up to serve both mother and baby, they contain equipment needed for the care and support of both. You will see equipment used by the anesthesia team. This includes machines to monitor you during the delivery, as well as others to provide oxygen or general anesthesia if needed. There will be carts with surgical instruments, drapes, and containers of various sizes. You will see the incubator or infant warmer ready to receive your baby. The pediatrics staff has a cart with supplies they need to clean and care for your infant. There is always resuscitation equipment available should you or your baby need it. In the midst of all of this is a very narrow table where the delivery will take place.

When you are first brought into the room there may be only a few members of the medical team present, but be assured the number will grow very quickly. There will be at least one nurse present, and often two or three. As the father in the birth report that begins this chapter pointed out, one of these nurses often acts as your "guide" for the birth. Her information and support can be invaluable to you during the preparation time and the delivery. The anesthesiologist and an assistant may be there when you arrive. There will be at least one person from the pediatric staff present, and possibly your own pediatrician will attend the birth. If you deliver at a teaching hospital, it is very likely that student nurses, an intern or two, and one or more residents will be in the room. The number can vary widely from hospital to hospital, but it will probably seem like a cast of thousands to you. All the equipment and all the people will be bathed in the lights necessary in any operating room. These often seem especially bright as they reflect against gleaming equipment and bare walls.

## ANESTHESIA

If you are going to have either spinal or epidural anesthesia, this will probably be given to you as soon as you enter the operating room. While you are waiting for it to take effect, the last-minute preparations for delivery will be completed. If you are to have a general, you will be completely prepared before the anesthesia is begun.

## GETTING YOU READY

You will be assisted from the rolling stretcher onto the operating table and asked to lie on your back. Most often the table is tilted slightly to keep the pressure of your uterus from falling directly on your major blood vessels and slowing your circulation. It is possible too that your right hip will be propped up slightly to aid circulation. If an IV was not started previously, it will be begun now. Also, if the catheter was not inserted before you were brought to the operating room, it will be put in place now. A blood pressure cuff will be loosely wrapped around one arm and, in many hospitals, discs for an EKG will be placed on your chest or near your shoulders. These rubber discs, which are attached to the EKG equipment, give the anesthesiologist a continuous check on your heart rate during delivery. It is entirely painless for you, but you may hear the "beeps" from the machine. These can be a bit disconcerting, especially since television has given many people a rather distorted impression of what the noises from an EKG mean.

Your abdomen and upper thighs will be thoroughly washed. They will then be "painted" or swabbed with an antiseptic solution. Both of these liquids are usually very cold. Hopefully, the nurse will warn you before she begins her work. Drapes will be placed over your abdomen, legs, and chest, so only the small area where the incision will be made is exposed. Your arms will be placed at your sides and gently restrained. Sometimes they are loosely strapped, sometimes wrapped in sheets. This is done so you do not inadvertently touch the sterile areas. Many times women request that one or both arms be left free. This request is often honored, especially if you want to hold your mate's hand or touch your baby right after delivery.

An anesthesia screen or drape will be put into place. This is set vertically so that you and the anesthesiologist will not contaminate the sterile field. The anesthesia drape prevents you from seeing the actual delivery. (If your mate is with you, he probably could see, if he just leaned out a bit.) Some hospitals provide mirrors so you can watch your baby being born if you wish. Sometimes the drape is lowered just as your baby is delivered. When such options are available, they are used only if you request them.

All of these things happen very quickly, and a number of procedures may be going on at the same time. The anesthesiologist may be testing to see if your regional anesthetic has taken effect yet. A nurse may be placing drapes over your body, and someone else may be putting a blood pressure cuff on your arm. There are times when the medical staff is so involved in getting your body ready for the delivery that they seem to forget your mind and your emotions, especially fear, which accompanied your body to this birth. If you begin to feel that only your abdomen is needed for this baby to be born, something is going wrong. Ask a question. Find someone to give you a running commentary on what is happening. Although the staff may see many babies being born every day, you will participate in only a few births, and these are very special moments for you.

When everything is ready, your obstetrician will join you. This is when your mate will be brought in if he is going to be with you. He will take his place near you, usually on a stool next to the anesthesiologist. As everyone gathers around you, you may feel as if you are surrounded by a sea of eyes, since everyone, including your mate, will be wearing a surgical mask.

## SKIN INCISIONS

There are two kinds of skin incisions that can be used for
Cesarean deliveries. Currently most women have a transverse or
"bikini" incision. (This is also called a Pfannenstiel incision.)
This is done very low on the abdomen, usually in the fold of the
lap just below the pubic hairline. The scar that results is usually
barely noticeable once it heals and the pubic hair grows back.

The second type, a vertical incision, runs from just below your
umbilicus down to the area of your pubic hair. It can be done
right in the middle of your abdomen (a midline incision), or a bit
to the side (a paramedian incision). In either case, it is certainly
more noticeable than a transverse incision, even though both
types of scars become less obvious with the passage of time.

Since the transverse skin incision is more acceptable to most
women, it is generally preferred. There are still cases when a vertical incision is used because it is thought to be faster to perform.
Even this is becoming less frequent, however, since with practice,
most doctors can perform a transverse skin incision with great
speed if necessary. There are still some doctors who are not experienced with "bikini" incisions and use a midline incision for all
Cesarean deliveries. This is something you should discuss with
your doctor early in your pregnancy.

## BEGINNING THE DELIVERY

First your skin is incised or cut. If you have had a previous surgical delivery, this skin incision will probably be the same as used
in the past. Also, if you have had a prior Cesarean, the scar
tissue will be removed so that you are left with only one scar.
Your skin will be retracted (pulled back and held with retractors) and your doctor will incise the subcutaneous tissue, the fatty

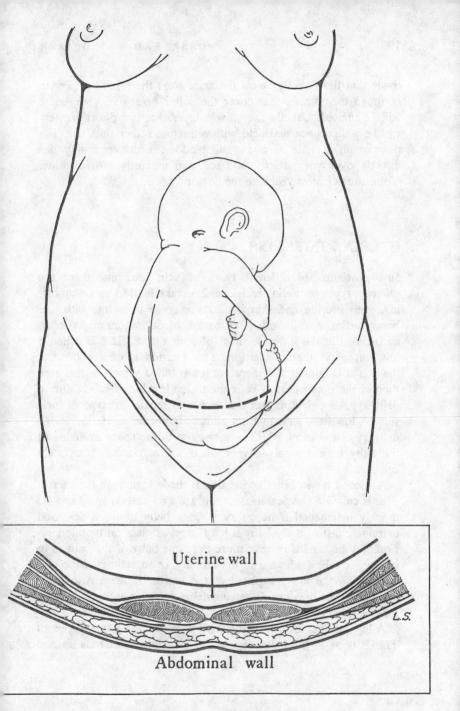

Uterine wall

Abdominal wall

*Skin Incision and Abdominal Layers*

tissue that lies directly below the skin. Next the fascia, the layers of tough membranes that cover the softer organs of your body, will be incised. Usually the muscle layer that lies directly below will be pulled back and held with retractors rather than cut. The peritoneum is entered and your bladder, which normally lies directly over your uterus, is freed and carefully moved aside. Your uterus is now visible to the doctor.

## UTERINE INCISIONS

Just as there are different types of skin incisions, there are different types of uterine incisions. To make matters more confusing, your uterine and skin incisions may be different, with one being vertical and the other horizontal. Most doctors prefer to do an incision in the lower segment of your uterus. This is called a low transverse uterine incision. This incision is chosen because the uterus is thinner and there are fewer blood vessels in this area than in the upper part of your uterus, so less blood is lost during delivery. Also, doctors feel it is easier to repair this type of incision. A low transverse incision allows about four to six inches for delivery of the baby, which is very close to the space available to the baby in a vaginal delivery when the cervix has completely opened.

A second type of uterine incision is made higher on the uterus. This is called a classical incision and runs up and down. It can be quickly lengthened if necessary when a baby must be delivered extremely fast or if the baby is very large. A classical uterine incision may be used if there is more than one baby, if the baby is in a transverse lie (sideways in the uterus), or sometimes if the placenta is in the lower segment of the uterus. If there is a lot of scarring from previous Cesarean deliveries, this type of incision may be done also.

A low vertical incision is the third type of uterine incision used. This is done in the lower segment of the uterus but runs up and down. It still minimizes blood loss and it can be extended when necessary. This kind of incision may be used if your doctor suspects that your baby is unusually large.

If this is a repeat Cesarean, you will probably have the same type of uterine incision used previously. Unless medically necessary, most doctors prefer to avoid intersecting uterine scars. There is a fear that the place where the two scars cross would be especially vulnerable to rupture.

## THE BIRTH

Your doctor will carefully incise your uterus. The amniotic fluid may gush out when this is done, or the doctor may have to gently rupture the amniotic sac. You will probably hear a suctioning noise as the amniotic fluid is removed.

The doctor then reaches in and carefully begins to remove your baby. If your baby is in the vertex (head down) position, her head will emerge first. If she is breech, a foot or the buttocks may be the first part to enter the world. Often the doctor or an assistant will push on the upper part of your uterus to help guide your baby through the relatively small opening made by the incision. If you have had regional anesthesia, it is very likely that you will feel some pressure and possibly tugging as your baby is lifted out. This can be momentarily disconcerting, but it means your baby is really here! Many women, especially if they are aware this may happen, feel a real sense of elation during this time.

Often the doctor will begin suctioning your baby as soon as the head is delivered. Suctioning will continue and the rest of the body will be gently pulled out. At times forceps are used, but this has become infrequent. If your baby's condition is good and the cord is long enough, your doctor may immediately hold the baby up so you can see and admire. You will hear that first cry, hear comments about the size of your baby, and finally have the answer to, "Is it a boy or a girl?"

Your baby's cord will be clamped and cut. Sometimes you get a very quick close-up view as the pediatric team whisks your baby to their work area. More often, it is possible to have your baby cleaned and evaluated quite near the operating table, even though your view may be partially blocked by the attending staff.

## FINISHING THE DELIVERY

While you are enjoying your first minutes of parenthood, many things will be happening. Your doctor will manually remove the placenta and examine your uterus for remaining placental tissue. Any remaining amniotic fluid will be suctioned out. Some doctors remove the uterus from the abdominal cavity so they can examine it more carefully and suture it more easily. If you have opted to have a sterilization procedure such as a tubal ligation done, or to have your appendix out, this will be done now.

Sometimes women feel dizzy or queasy right after delivery. This is usually because of the sudden change in uterine pressure as the baby is delivered. Most often it can be corrected by giving you oxygen for a few minutes. Or, medications may be given which relieve nausea. At times, the discomfort is more extreme, and medication will be given so you sleep while suturing is being done. Some doctors routinely give a sleeping medication through the IV once your baby is born. Make sure you tell your doctor if you prefer not to have this kind of medication. Many women would rather be awake for the suturing so they will be sure to be alert during their time in the recovery room, especially if the baby will be brought to them there.

You may feel that the rest is anticlimax, but the surgical team has completed only a small part of its work. From the start of surgery until the birth of your baby, only about three to seven minutes have gone by. Approximately thirty to forty-five minutes (some doctors take longer) will be needed to complete the repairs.

Just as the delivery was carefully done layer by layer, so too is the repair accomplished. Each uterine layer is individually stitched. Your bladder is returned to its normal position and stitched into place. Each internal layer is separately sutured, usually with a dissolvable material. Your doctor carefully cleans out the abdominal cavity and checks for any bleeding. Finally, the skin incision is closed. This is often done with one continuous suture, rather than interrupted stitches, so a better-looking scar will result. Either dissolvable or nondissolvable material may be used. (If nondissolvable sutures are put in, they will be removed before you leave the hospital.) Some doctors use clamps or adhesive materials rather than sutures. In all you will have about six or seven separate layers of stitches, of which you see only one. That terrible fear that occurs to many women, that they may just split back open, is really not likely to occur—even if you cough!

All during this time, your pulse and general condition will be watched carefully. Before you are taken to the recovery room, you may have a chance to see your baby once more. Even better, your husband, your baby, and you may all go to the recovery room together and have an immediate start on becoming a family.

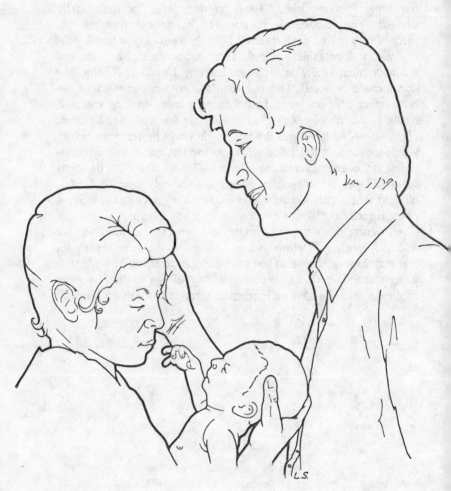

*The New Family*

## SEVEN

# Your Baby's First Week of Life

## WELCOME TO THE WORLD

The baby is born at last! In just a few short minutes, your pregnancy has ended and a new, separate person has come into your lives.

> I felt an overwhelming sense of joy at that moment when I first heard the baby cry. The doctor said, "We've got the head—we've got the shoulders—it's a boy!" and I felt the happiest moment I've ever known. It's that moment that reconnected me with all the women of whom I'd been so bitterly envious, the women who could deliver vaginally. I felt that *they* should envy *me*, for without having gone through the loneliness, the anxiety, and the fears that I'd had, they could never feel that contrasting joy as intensely as I felt it. My disappointments virtually vanished.

The cord is clamped and then your doctor will hand the baby to the nurse or pediatrician who is standing by. If you have had a regional anesthetic, and if you are not exhausted from the strain of a long labor, you may be an eager observer in these first few

minutes of your baby's life. The baby will be suctioned and evaluated, probably by two people simultaneously, so you may not be
able to see much even if the baby's care is done within your field
of vision. Hopefully, the people who are caring for the baby will
bring him to you for a closer look, and you will be able to touch
him once the preliminary evaluation is completed.

As a rule, Cesarean babies tend to be "prettier" than those who
were delivered vaginally. This is because the baby's head has not
been as molded and squeezed by the passage through the birth
canal. In other respects, the baby will look about the same as babies who are delivered vaginally. He may have some *vernix,* the
greasy coating that protected his skin when he was in the uterus,
still remaining. He probably will also have some of the long hair
called *lanugo,* which can appear all over the body of a newborn.
If the baby has not been completely cleaned up, you may see
some fluid that looks like blood, but that is mostly amniotic fluid
with a little blood mixed in. If the baby has been completely
dried off before you see him, you may simply notice the slight
bluish tinge of his hands and feet. This, too, is characteristic of
many newborns, and has no relationship to how your baby came
into the world.

> When they showed him to me, I started to cry and laugh all at
> once. I remember saying, "It's Jonathan; hello, Jonathan!" and
> laughing and crying for joy. He was the most beautiful baby I had
> ever seen.

## EVALUATION AND ROUTINE BABY CARE

The main medical tasks at this point are to clear the baby's airway (mouth, nose, and throat), to keep him warm, and to be sure
that his condition is good. As part of this process, doctors use a
system of assessment called the Apgar score. A look at the chart
below will show you how the baby's Apgar score is determined.
There are five indicators that are measured, and the baby may
receive a score from 0 to 2 on each indicator. This means that the

highest possible score is 10, although a perfect score is unusual. The system of Apgar scores allows your doctor to make a rapid judgment of your baby's condition using objectively tested criteria. (This system is used to evaluate all babies, whether delivered vaginally or by Cesarean.) Apgar scores are determined when the baby is one minute old and again when he is five minutes old. Most babies score 8 or 9. Scores between 4 and 7 indicate that the baby has some problem, although it may not be a serious one. Immediate steps will be taken to evaluate the baby further and to treat him. A score of less than 4 means that the baby has a serious problem. The Apgar system is only one of the methods that your pediatrician has for evaluating your baby. The scores are guidelines, not absolute measures of your baby's health. (If your baby had some problem at birth, or if you have some condition that leads you to expect such problems, please turn to Chapter Twelve, "When Something Goes Wrong.")

## HOW THE APGAR SCORE IS DETERMINED

| SIGN | SCORE 0 | SCORE 1 | SCORE 2 |
|---|---|---|---|
| Heartbeat | Absent | Less than 100 beats per minute | More than 100 beats per minute |
| Respiratory Effort | Absent | Shallow, gasping, weak cry | Vigorous, sustained, lusty cry |
| Reflex Irritability* | Absent | Frown, grimace | Grimace, sneezing, coughing, crying |
| Muscle Tone | Limp | Some flexing of arms and legs | Active motion, arms and legs well flexed |
| Color | Blue, pale | Body pink, arms and legs blue | Entirely pink |

* Response to flick of finger against foot or catheter inserted into nostril.

The suctioning of the baby's airway, which may have begun when his head was delivered but before he was removed from your uterus, continues now. In addition, it is not unusual for oxygen to be administered to the baby. Cesarean babies tend to have more mucus and fluids remaining in their lungs and breathing passages at birth. Apparently, the advantage to the baby of feeling the big squeeze of vaginal birth is that these fluids are pushed out and the baby's respiratory system is given that emphatic signal to take over.

The staff who are caring for your baby will be careful to maintain his body temperature, usually by placing him in a warmer unit while he is being suctioned and evaluated. Sometimes a heat-sensitive detector is taped to the baby's skin. Keeping the baby in the warmer or keeping him wrapped insures that he will maintain enough body heat to keep his metabolic system functioning normally.

Several additional procedures must be completed before the baby is taken to the nursery. Identification bands are attached to the baby's wrist or ankle. Sometimes footprints are taken at this time. There will certainly be no doubt that this is the right baby!

Most hospitals choose this time to administer silver nitrate or penicillin to the baby's eyes. This is required by law in all states, to prevent possible blindness caused by gonorrhea bacteria. Actually, Cesarean babies are not usually exposed to these bacteria, which are found in the vaginal canal. Silver nitrate usually causes some swelling and irritation of the eyelids for a few days. Penicillin is less irritating, but also less effective. You may ask that it not be given immediately, although at least one state law requires that it be administered at birth without delay.

## OTHER POSSIBLE PROCEDURES

A variety of other procedures may be carried out now, depending simply on whether that is your hospital's way of doing things. In some hospitals, the baby's heel is pricked and a small sample of blood drawn. This blood is tested to make sure the baby is not anemic and to determine whether he is Rh positive or negative. Some doctors prefer to use blood from the umbilical cord for this purpose. In addition, the baby will be tested for the disease called PKU, through blood drawn in the next few days. PKU is a rare inherited disease that can be treated if detected early but that causes brain damage if it goes unnoticed for long.

Some hospitals also give babies an injection of vitamin K, which is thought to help prevent bleeding.

## GETTING THE FAMILY TOGETHER

Once the baby has been completely examined and his temperature has been stabilized, he traditionally is taken to the nursery for further care and observation. However, some hospitals are encouraging parents to have a quiet time alone with their baby in the recovery room before the mother returns to her room and the baby goes to the nursery. Most hospitals still do not permit fathers to be present for a Cesarean birth, but the hospital administration may have no objection to a compromise first meeting in the recovery room. In order for this to be feasible, your hospital must have their Cesarean births performed in the maternity area so that the recovery room is not also occupied by other surgical patients.

In some hospitals, Cesarean babies are routinely taken to the special care nursery for the first twenty-four hours. This policy is a leftover from the days when a Cesarean was really a last resort, performed in a desperate attempt to save mother and baby. The likelihood that the baby would have complications then was high, and the close observation afforded by the intensive care nursery was only sensible. Currently, fewer hospitals automatically place all Cesarean babies in the intensive care nursery. The decision is most often made on the basis of the individual infant's needs.

If your baby does go to an intensive care nursery simply because that is hospital policy, there may be some unexpected benefits for other family members. You probably will not be up to caring for the baby in these first twenty-four hours, but the baby may be brought to your room for brief visits, especially if you or your husband ask persistently. As soon as you are able to get out of bed, you may visit the nursery. You may be more comfortable making the trip in a wheelchair, especially if the nursery is any distance from your room. In the meantime, we know of at least one hospital where grandparents were invited in to the special care nursery to hold and feed the baby, while they would have been kept standing behind a glass observation window if the baby had been in the regular nursery.

In any case, if your husband has not been allowed to be with you for the birth of the baby and has not been able to join you in the recovery room, then his first introduction to the baby will probably be when the baby is being taken to the nursery. In fact, he may be invited to come along and get acquainted while you are still being stitched.

I know I only waited a few minutes, but it seemed like forever. I suddenly got scared that something had really gone wrong, but there was the nurse at last, holding this screaming bundle wrapped in a yellow blanket. For a split second I thought, "Yellow? How am I supposed to know if it's a boy or a girl?" and then she said, "You have a fine, healthy son." I remembered to ask how much he weighed, and then the nurse said I could hold him, and I got really nervous. But I did sit down and she showed me how to hold him. The amazing thing is that he stopped crying then. I've never forgotten that moment.

## NURSERY ROUTINES

Once he arrives in the nursery, your baby's care is determined by his condition and by your hospital's usual practices. These vary widely, although they are all designed to accomplish the same goals. The hospital staff continues to take measures to maintain the baby's body temperature. In the intensive care nursery, the baby may be in an isolette with an individual temperature control. In the regular nursery, he may simply be dressed or wrapped in blankets. Because humans lose so much body heat from their scalp, some hospitals have started putting little knitted caps on the newborns.

The concern about the baby's airway remaining clear continues, and some hospitals place Cesarean babies in a slightly tilted-down position to encourage further drainage of fluids. Some of the medications that are given to women in labor may contribute further to the problem, since they seem to weaken the baby's reflexes somewhat. This means that he may not cough up mucus as effectively as a baby whose mother had no medication during delivery. Occasionally, additional suctioning of fluids will be done after the baby goes to the nursery.

## FIRST PHYSICAL EXAMINATION

Sometime during the first day your baby will have a complete physical examination. If you have chosen a pediatric group, there may be one member of that group who does all of the newborn physicals for the entire group. Or your regular pediatrician may do the physical. If you have a family physician who does not do physicals in the hospital, then the exam will be done by a regular member of the hospital pediatric staff. You may wish to be present when the physical is done, and there is probably no reason why you cannot, as long as you are feeling up to it. The doctor may be willing to perform the examination in your room, for your comfort. Be sure to let both your pediatrician and the nurses in the nursery know if you want to observe.

> The doctor was so thorough. I was amazed at how many things she could check on such a tiny baby. When she saw how interested I was, she explained everything as she did it. I like that and it gave me even more confidence that I had chosen the right doctor.

## GETTING TO KNOW THE BABY

You may have planned to take advantage of your hospital's policy of rooming-in—that is, keeping the baby in your room, instead of having him remain in the nursery between feedings. Having a Cesarean birth will interfere with your plans somewhat, although you may still have the baby with you much of the time if the hospital policy is flexible. During the first day or two, you will need your husband or another helper with you while the baby is in the room. This is the person who can bring the baby to you, hold him while you change positions or adjust the bed to a more comfortable level, and do the necessary lifting and bending when diapers must be changed. Usually, all of the equipment you need will be stored in a small cabinet in the baby's rolling crib.

Your baby may seem bored with the proceedings, and sleep through most of the day. This can be restful, but boring, for you too. If the baby is the sleepy type, then rooming-in may appeal to you even more, since it increases your chances to enjoy the short periods when the baby is alert.

Most babies alternate sleep with some wakefulness and perhaps long periods of being restless or full of complaints. If yours is an active baby, then modified rooming-in may be a better arrangement for you. This system allows you to return the baby to the skilled hands of the nursery nurses whenever his demands exceed your resources. Even a relatively quiet baby may have the knack of waking up just as you start to doze, so flexibility and taking care of yourself are the keys to getting a good start with the baby.

I never changed a diaper before in my life. But my wife said that she hadn't changed one in more than fifteen years, so she couldn't see how that was any excuse. It was obvious that she couldn't hop out of bed and rescue me, so I just went ahead and did it. The hospital used disposable diapers, and I thought I was doing really great for a new Dad. Later, the nurse came in and noticed the diaper was backward. Well, I may not be perfect, but it worked fine the way I did it. I also make better spaghetti sauce than anyone in town!

# FEEDING YOUR BABY

## Which Way?

By the time you learned that you definitely were going to have a Cesarean, you probably had already decided on the method of feeding that seemed best for you. If you want to breast-feed your baby, having a Cesarean delivery may complicate the picture somewhat, but a few adjustments on your part will take care of any problems that arise. Occasionally, parents are told that Cesarean mothers cannot successfully nurse their babies. This is completely untrue, although being surrounded by people who have such a negative attitude may contribute to a mother's difficulties. Some women who have a Cesarean become even more determined to succeed at breast-feeding than they were when they expected a vaginal delivery.

> I felt like such a failure because of the Cesarean. But I said to myself, "Maybe I can't have the baby all by myself, but I damn sure can feed her." When my milk came in I felt so good. I think I could have nursed twins. It made up for so much that I felt I had missed.

Nursing has benefits for both mother and baby. For the baby, there is evidence that colostrum, which is secreted from the breasts before breast milk appears, provides important protection from diseases that formula does not. For the mother, the uterine contractions that occur when the baby nurses are beneficial in helping the uterus to return to normal size. From an emotional standpoint, the rewards of nursing for both mother and baby may be even greater when the birth is by Cesarean.

For various reasons, parents may choose to give the baby formula. The most important issue for you as a parent is whether you feel comfortable with the decision you have made. Although the American Academy of Pediatrics states that breast milk is "the best food for every newborn infant," you may have needs as a parent that make bottle-feeding the best choice for you.

> I was pretty sure I didn't want to nurse the baby. My husband was against it. I would be going back to work so soon. Even though my pregnancy was an accident and the timing couldn't have been worse, we were looking forward to this birth. But there was no way I could be the perfect mother like some of the magazines pictured.

### Successful Nursing

If you are convinced that you want to breast-feed your baby, then you are very likely to be successful. Many good books on the subject are available, but the best help comes from mothers who have already done it, or nurses who take the time and have the experience to help you get past whatever hurdles may develop. Here are some hints that will help you to have a better nursing experience.

1. *Arrange to have modified rooming-in* as soon as you feel ready. No matter how the baby was born, successful breast-feeding involves you and the baby establishing a close relationship based on mutual need.

2. *Rest!* This will be no problem in the beginning. But many Cesarean mothers are feeling so comfortable and so elated about the baby's birth by the third or fourth postpartum day that they make the mistake of overdoing it. A little activity each hour of the day will be much better for you than pushing yourself to your limits before lunch is served.

3. *Drink plenty of fluids,* especially water and fruit juices. They will help your gastrointestinal tract to return to normal, so that you can resume a regular diet. In addition, they are essential simply because your body loses so much fluid when the baby nurses. You should continue to drink extra fluids as long as you nurse the baby.

4. *Ask for help.* In some hospitals, the nurses know just the

right thing to suggest when you have a question. Sometimes the best helper is another mother who has nursed or is nursing a baby. The La Leche League will visit mothers in the hospital if you need help.

5. *Relax.* Breast-feeding doesn't come instinctively to anyone. Like good sex, it is a natural function that also must be learned in order to be enjoyed to its fullest. Part of the learning for you will be getting to know this particular baby. Each baby is different in his need to suck, his willingness to pay attention while nursing, etc.

6. *Try different positions.* You may find it easiest at first to take the baby into bed with you, with the head of the bed mostly raised; then lie so that you are turned slightly toward the baby as he rests next to you, held in the crook of your arm. As they begin to feel better, some women like to sit cross-legged in bed with the raised head for support, a pillow or two behind them, and one in their lap under the baby. Or ask the nurses to show you the "football carry," which involves holding the baby against your side with his feet extended behind you. In this position, the baby is supported by pillows and does not rest on your tender abdomen.

7. *Enlist your obstetrician's and pediatrician's support.* There may be hospital rules that, although they are meant to help you, actually interfere with nursing. For instance, the hospital may encourage feeding on demand during the day, but keep the baby on a strict schedule during the night because "Cesarean mothers need their rest." Yet your milk may be better established if you feed the baby on demand at night too, to the extent that you feel up to it. Probably the best way to get around these kinds of policies is to ask the doctor to leave orders that you may have the baby more frequently if you wish.

8. *Be patient.* Mothers and babies are often out of phase with each other in this early stage of nursing. You may have very full and uncomfortable breasts, and a baby who wants to sleep rather than eat. Or you may be the one wishing for a nap, while the baby just wants to keep nursing for the rest of his life. And the

fact that you have so little strength at this time makes these differences between you harder to cope with.

> I felt just frantic to get my hands on that baby. It just didn't seem right to go through all that and then not have a baby in my arms. But when they brought her in, I realized that I was a cripple compared to my roommate. I couldn't even get out of bed and take her from the nurse. So I had my baby at last, but I didn't know what to do with her. The nurse got the head of the bed raised up and showed me how to prop myself up and hold her. We finally got both of us arranged, and then she wasn't even interested in nursing. She got the nipple partly into her mouth and fell asleep. The nurse didn't seem too surprised, and she just said we would try again later in the morning. She took the baby back to the nursery, and I got my pain shot and fell asleep. Maybe the rest did us both some good, because the next time it went better.

9. *Be flexible.* This is no time for the purist approach to anything. You may have planned to nurse the baby exclusively, avoiding any supplementary bottles of formula, water, or sugar water, and many Cesarean mothers are able to do this. But your success at nursing after a Cesarean depends on your taking good care of yourself. You should nurse the baby as often as he wants, as long as you feel comfortable doing so. But in spite of what you may have read or been told, an occasional bottle will not interfere with successful nursing for most babies. And an uninterrupted night's sleep, with your husband or the nurses giving the baby a bottle, may be just the thing you need to start feeling on top of life again.

### Breast-feeding Through Separation
Occasionally, either mother or baby develops some complication that results in a separation. If the baby has a condition that requires him to remain in the special care nursery, then you will begin nursing without the benefits of a comfortable bed. The staff will help you get to the nursery in a wheelchair until the third or fourth day, when you are able to walk. Be sure to take along a pillow to place on your lap while you are nursing. There may be a quiet corner and even a rocking chair where you and the baby can get started together.

Sometimes it is possible to avoid separation with a little creativity and special consideration from the hospital staff. One Cesarean mother was told that her baby had to remain in the special care nursery under some lights because the baby was jaundiced. She asked to have both the baby and the lights moved to her room. This was unheard of, and the woman might never have thought to ask, except that she was also employed as a nurse on that very floor! Her request was granted when the staff considered it carefully and could find no reason to say no. Then the staff began to question why all mothers in these circumstances could not have the same privilege.

Sometimes a baby has needs that are best cared for in another hospital. Or his hospital stay may be prolonged, even though you are released to go home. This kind of separation makes breastfeeding much more difficult. Even so, it can be done, especially if the separation will be relatively brief. It will be necessary to express your milk, a trick that some women find is a cinch and others really struggle with. A breast pump may help. The simplest kind sold in drugstores is adequate for a few women, while others use the more sophisticated pumps that your hospital or the local La Leche League may make available. The hospital staff will help you, and will store the breast milk in the refrigerator or freezer until it is used or transported.

If the baby must remain in the hospital for an extended period, then your success at continuing to nurse the baby will be determined to some extent by what is going on in the rest of your life. In addition to dedication, it helps to have help with other children, no plans to go back to work or school, and a supportive husband. If it does become necessary to wean the baby, you may experience some relief from the stress of the effort you were making, as well as regret that you are unable to continue. You may be reassured that the baby has benefited from your getting this far.

### What About Medication?
One of the biggest concerns that Cesarean mothers who nurse their babies face is the question of how the pain medication that they need during the early recovery period will affect the baby. Most doctors and groups that support breast-feeding are very re-

assuring in their answers. They usually say that the types of medications that mothers take and the quantities that reach the baby through the milk are not harmful to the baby. It is true that the available evidence, both from research and firsthand experience, suggests that it is both safe and advisable for Cesarean mothers to breast-feed. There are millions of healthy children whose mothers had a Cesarean and then nursed them. However, this is not the same as saying that there is proof that it is safe to take the medications and breast-feed your baby. What is true is that conclusive data based on valid research are not available, even with regard to short-term effects on babies. Even if extensive studies were undertaken immediately, the data regarding long range effects of medication would not be available for many years.

The assumptions about the safety of pain medication for breast-feeding Cesarean mothers are widespread. They have come about partly because professionals and consumers who support nursing mothers know that it is virtually impossible to recover from a Cesarean without using some medication. Therefore, when evidence that supports the safety of these drugs is produced, it may be accepted with relief rather than challenged. Additionally, most professionals and lay groups rely on readily available, easily readable "review articles" that summarize a large number of individual drug studies. Unfortunately, many of these original studies may be so old, or their study design so poorly constructed that their conclusions would be seen as unacceptable by many experts in pharmacological research. Although this is a highly technical subject, the various complaints about the original research are easily summarized:

A) Drug manufacturers' unpublished data are reported without any description of how the results were obtained. Since drug manufacturers naturally want to believe their products are safe, it is essential that their studies be scrutinized to ensure that the results are not biased by the way in which the studies are conducted.

B) Animal data are used to imply that a drug is safe for humans. In fact, there are no animal models that duplicate human lactation and infant response.

C) Older research is reported, going as far back as the 1930s. Techniques for measuring the presence of a drug in breast milk at that time were quite primitive, so it is entirely possible that its presence was undetected. Studies that utilize current technology must be undertaken in order to re-examine the effects of drugs that have been commonly used for many years.

D) A very small number of mothers are tested—sometimes only one—yet the results are reported as though they were valid for many. There is a great deal of individual variation in how mothers and infants respond to a given drug.

E) Only one dose of a drug is given, although in clinical practice the drug would be administered repeatedly.

F) The levels of the drug are measured infrequently or in random fashion, without regard to when the drug was administered. Drug milk levels may be less than, equal to, or greater than blood levels, with a peak level (highest concentration) and valley level (lowest concentration) that can vary greatly. The timing and extent of peak and valley levels depend on the drug, amount given, time and frequency of dose, and many other factors. Breast milk must be tested at numerous specific intervals, not a few times or randomly, to get a true picture.

G) Studies ignore the importance of the stage of breast-feeding (colostrum, early infancy, premature baby, or older infant) as well as the time of day and duration of feedings. This is important because colostrum, which is excreted by the mother during the first few days after birth, is low in fat but high in some electrolytes. Mothers of premature babies have milk that is chemically different from those of full-term babies. The ratio of fat to electrolytes also changes as the baby matures. The amount of fat in the milk is also influenced by the time of day (highest fat levels at midmorning) and the duration of feeding (toward the end of each feeding, the fat content is higher). Both fat content and electrolytes may influence the concentration of some drugs.

H) Some review articles cite results from other review articles, with the result that information is carried forward from one article to the next. The original research or speculation that is being referred to is often no longer available, so it may be difficult or impossible to determine how the data were acquired. There is the additional danger that speculation can grow to the status of truth, accumulating new weight each time it is cited.

I) There is no research on drugs in colostrum, although the period when colostrum is excreted is also the period when Cesarean mothers most need medication for pain. Yet colostrum contains the immunoglobulins, which are so valuable to the baby in providing protection from disease.

If you want to nurse your baby, there are a few things you can do that may help you to avoid some of the potential risks associated with your taking pain medication. One is to ask your doctor to discuss your concerns with you. His or her choice of the most appropriate drug for you is not easy in light of the lack of definitive information, but there are choices to be made. Of several drugs in the same pharmacological category, one may be more suitable than the other for you as a breast-feeding mother, and for your baby.

Another help may be to nurse the baby immediately before or immediately after you have taken an oral medication, or immediately before if the medication is given by injection. Although the data are unclear on this point, it seems likely from a theoretical standpoint that the level of medication in your milk will be lower at these times. Since it is best to breast-feed whenever the baby wants to nurse, you may have to adjust your own schedule of medication somewhat in order to manage this. It is wise to use as low a dose of the medication as possible, and to prolong the intervals between doses. Using relaxation techniques, playing with the baby, or finding something else to divert your attention from your pain may be helpful, especially when used in combination with medication. It is not necessary for you to take a pill simply because it is offered. On the other hand, it would be senseless to refuse medication when you really need it. Your comfort and ability to cope with your situation are essential for your own recovery and for your ability to establish a good nursing relationship with your baby.

Babies who are unusually sleepy, irritable, or who exhibit vomiting or diarrhea may be showing signs of being hypersensitive to your medication. If your baby has problems after birth, you should request that your pediatrician consider the possibility that your medication may be making a contribution to the baby's condition.

> I really wanted to breast-feed the baby. Since I read a lot, I knew that there are chemicals in the environment that get into mothers' milk. My doctor tried to reassure me, but when I asked more questions he backed off and said they really don't know all there is to know about the problem. Then came the Cesarean, and the story was the same: We don't think your medicine affects the baby, but we are not 100 per cent sure. I do OK when I have the facts, even unpleasant facts. But all these unknowns really threw us both. It shouldn't be so hard to do the right thing! In the end, we shrugged off our doubts and I nursed her. I've always been glad.

## THIS BABY—THIS MIRACLE

What is life like for the baby in the first week? Most parents have heard that their newborn baby cannot see and does not take in his surroundings very much. However, the most recent studies have demonstrated that we have greatly underestimated the capacity of newborn babies to take in and respond to their new world.

Researchers who have studied newborns have distinguished six categories of behavior that babies exhibit. In the first, the baby is sleeping soundly and breathing regularly. The second is described as light sleep and occasional restlessness, with irregular breathing. The third category is when the baby is simply drowsy, and the fourth is called the quiet, alert state. Next, there is the alert and actively moving state, and the final category is when the baby is crying.

Scientists have become fascinated with the elusive fourth state, when the baby is most responsive to the world around him. It is "elusive" because few babies remain quiet and alert for long periods of time in their early weeks. A newborn baby may exhibit the characteristics of the fourth state for just a few seconds or moments at a time, although the amounts of time that he is quiet and alert will increase with each week of life.

By closely observing babies in the quiet, alert state, scientists have discovered that newborns are sometimes exquisitely sensitive creatures. Your baby can see best at a distance of about ten inches. He will show a definite preference, through his movements and facial expressions, for objects that have sharp contrast as opposed to dull gray. Even at four days old, your baby will look more at a picture of a human face and less at a picture of a face with the features in the wrong place. At two weeks, your baby will look much more at your face, and will look away from a stranger.

There is no doubt that babies can hear while they are in the uterus. Your baby will continue to hear and respond to sound in complicated ways in the days right after birth. For instance, if you speak, the baby will search around for the source of your voice. It has even been demonstrated, through frame-by-frame analysis of films of newborns, that their movements are synchronized with human speech. If you have seen any of the new slow-motion films of parents and babies right after birth, then you know that babies in the quiet, alert state seem to be carrying on a dialogue with their parents.

Babies also have well-developed senses of smell, taste, and touch. Six-day-old babies can distinguish between their mother's breastpads and those of another breast-feeding mother. Some babies will vigorously refuse water, and even glucose water, after several days of being fed breast milk or formula. Probably the most startling new observation of all was again discovered by frame-by-frame analysis of films of newborns: They imitate the facial expressions of adults. What a far cry this is from the things our mothers taught us!

Certainly the baby is not this sensitive all the time. In fact, he will spend most of his early days sleeping, and, of course, crying.

Babies seem to have periods of disorganization in these first few days of life, followed by periods of leveling off. When they get older, you can recognize the "growth spurts" and learn how to respond to them. But at this early age, these times seem like a bewildering phase where nothing goes right for the baby, and nothing you do seems right either. The baby may want to suck a lot, even when you feel pretty sure he is not hungry. He may fuss or even cry hard when you know that he is dry, not too warm or too cold, not bothered by bright lights or startling noises. Sometimes the rhythm of being rocked or walked about will soothe him. But you may not feel ready to cope with the baby's needs at a time when you are feeling pretty needy too. Even if you want nothing more than the chance to mother him, you may simply not have the physical strength to walk the floors. Your husband or the hospital staff should take over now, while you rest and take care of yourself.

By the time you are ready to go home from the hospital, you probably will have some hints about what kind of baby this is. He will seem "easy" or "active" and you will begin adjusting to the ways in which he is different from what you expected and different from your other children, or your sister's, or the kind of baby you were.

At first I couldn't get them to let me have the baby. I was a section mother, so they didn't think I was up to it. Then my fever went up for a day and the baby couldn't come to my room then either. It was almost three days before they brought him to me. I didn't feel right about him until we got home and I could have him to myself. I would sit and rock him, and sing any little song that came to me. Sometimes he seemed to take it all in. Sometimes he just snuggled in my arms and went to sleep. I would just keep holding him and rocking him. That was when we had our beginning together.

# EIGHT

# Your Early Recovery

## FIRST TWENTY-FOUR HOURS

### Immediate Concerns

Now that your baby is born, your concern quite naturally turns to yourself. You may be quite alert during the time right after the birth, or you may feel very sleepy, particularly if you have had a long labor.

> I remember the Apgar scores. The first was 8 and the second, 9. I remember that Jack was with me for a while in the recovery room. The nurses kept coming in and waking me up. It seemed like I would just be dozing off and someone would come in again. I don't know what they were doing there. It is all such a blur in my mind.

Part of your feelings during this early recovery period will reflect your surroundings. If your hospital does Cesarean births on the maternity floor, then the recovery room is a happy place where births are often celebrated. You may be the only person being cared for, or one of just a few. If you have had regional anesthesia, you may remain quite comfortable for a short time, and enjoy a visit with your baby and your husband.

> They brought her in, and she looked so little, but wonderful. I kept telling her what her name was, and saying silly things, until she finally looked at me. Ron seemed so excited. He asked me if I was all right, and I remember saying I was just *fine*.

In some hospitals, Cesareans are performed in the general surgery area. In this case, the recovery room will be occupied by patients in different stages of recovery from all kinds of surgery. Neither your husband nor your baby will be allowed to visit you, and the nurses who are caring for you will not be the ones you got to know if you were in labor. This can be a difficult time, although for some women the joy of the baby's birth is so great that the question of where they are recovering is immaterial.

Your stay in the recovery room may be as short as an hour or two or as long as all night. This depends partly on the speed of your recovery, but it also depends on such matters as how busy the regular maternity floor is. Some hospitals do not transfer anyone out of recovery during the midnight shift.

### As the Anesthesia Wears Off

If you have had a general anesthetic, you probably will remain very groggy in the immediate postoperative period. You may wake up and talk with those around you for a few minutes, then fall asleep again and wake up with no concept of how much time has passed. In retrospect, this may seem like a continuously painful time, since you will remember your wakeful times and not the periods in between when you were sleeping. General anesthesia lingers in your body for a while, and pain medication is available when it has subsided and you are aware of the discomfort. You may already have received some medication for pain during surgery, after the baby was born.

If you have had a spinal, you may be required to lie flat on your back for the next twenty-four hours. Until recently, this was thought to prevent spinal headaches. Many doctors now agree that remaining on your back is helpful if a headache actually occurs, but not as a prevention. For some women, the restriction against sitting up seems like no restriction at all, since they have very little inclination to start moving around. The paralysis and absence of sensation caused by the spinal may continue for several hours, although it is more common for it to begin to wear off soon after you go to the recovery room. The wearing off starts with a sensation of warmth and tingling, usually beginning with the feet, which some women find very odd. The nurse will ask you to wiggle your toes, but many women find they cannot manage this on the first few tries. Gradually the message will travel all the way from your brain to your feet, and you will regain feeling and the ability to move.

If you have had an epidural anesthetic, you may go to the recovery room with the anesthesia tube still in place. Some doctors choose to continue administering epidural anesthetic during the early recovery period, to help you get past the worst discomfort. If you have had an epidural, you will not have experienced any paralysis. You will regain full sensation not long after the anesthesia is discontinued.

The early recovery period is quite tolerable to some women, and just plain awful for others. The variation in the amount of pain that women report is due to many factors, including the amount and kind of anesthesia and medications used, the unique response of your body to surgery and anesthesia, and the extent to which your exhilaration about the baby masks the pain. In any case, pain medication has been ordered for you, usually starting when abdominal sensation has returned, and it will be very helpful at this time. It will be given in the form of an injection, since you are not permitted to take anything by mouth. To the extent that you do feel pain, it can come from three separate sources. Obviously, the site of the incision is the main one. In addition, your uterus is contracting, and this can add to the discomfort. Some mothers also feel pain under the shoulder blade, which can be caused by air trapped under their diaphragm during the birth.

Occasionally doctors prescribe tranquilizers at this time too. They are meant to help you get over any anxiety or upset feelings you may be having about the birth and the baby. Although tranquilizers may be helpful to some, the main effect they have for most women is simply to postpone dealing with the feelings about the birth. If your Cesarean is a planned event, you may want to share your preferences about this with your doctor.

### Things the Nurses Do for You

The nurses will be very busy during this time, checking your pulse, respiration, and blood pressure. They will also look at the area of the incision, and they will examine your vaginal area and peripad (a large sanitary napkin) to see how much vaginal bleeding is occurring. The purpose of all this is to make sure that your postoperative recovery is normal and that you are not experiencing too much bleeding. In addition, the nurses will examine your abdomen to determine the height of your uterus, and they will press on your abdomen in order to put pressure on the top part of the uterus (fundus). This procedure is very uncomfortable, but it is very important. It pushes the accumulated blood out of the vagina and encourages the uterus to contract.

During this recovery room period and for a day or two after the baby's birth, you will remain attached to various tubes and pieces of equipment. The catheter is one of these, and the nurses will check the catheter bag and empty and measure its contents periodically. During surgery, the bladder was moved from its normal position in front of your uterus, then stitched back into place after the baby was born. This necessary process causes some trauma to your bladder. The shock of surgery also diminishes all your bodily functions, including your ability to urinate. This is one reason your urine production is such a concern at this time.

The IV that was inserted prior to the birth becomes significant during the early recovery period for a new reason. Most doctors add some form of oxytocic drug to the IV, just as they do for women who have delivered vaginally. The purpose of this medication is to stimulate postpartum contractions of the uterus, which help minimize bleeding. Unfortunately, these contractions can add a great deal to your discomfort during the early part of the recovery period. If you can gather your forces of concentration enough to do some of the breathing exercises taught in your childbirth preparation class, you may feel more comfortable. If you feel a sensation something like a very strong or continuous contraction, you should ask to have the IV checked. The oxytocic drug will usually be discontinued after four to six hours. Your uterus will continue to contract on its own for a while after the medication has been discontinued.

In many hospitals, a sponge bath is given while you are in the recovery room. An experienced nurse can bathe you in a way that feels very refreshing, without adding to your discomfort. It does hurt more when you move than it does if you lie still. However, moving will hasten your recovery, so this is a good time to get started. The nurse will help you turn over, one step at a time. This seems like a major achievement now, but soon you will be moving around freely again.

If you are experiencing a very dry mouth, you may ask for some lemon-flavored swabs. You can wipe away some of the bad taste from your mouth and gums before you are allowed water.

You may rest most comfortably on your side, with pillows adding support. For many women, the greatest comfort is found in the following position: As you turn to lie on your side, ask the nurse to place pillows firmly against your back to keep you from rolling over. Bend your underneath leg to a comfortable angle. Then support the top leg by placing one or two pillows underneath it at the knee and wherever they feel comfortable, so that the top leg is slightly more bent and a little forward of the bottom leg. Then arrange your arms in whatever way seems most comfortable. The nurse will place the catheter bag appropriately and untangle the sheets as you change positions.

At the time it was happening, I was only thinking about the baby. I remember when the shift changed and I got new nurses, so I had a fresh audience. I told them all how she was the first girl born into the whole family in this generation, and how she has seven boy cousins. But now that I am pregnant again, I keep thinking how helpless I was then. Truthfully, I kind of dread it, but I know it's unavoidable. I try to reassure myself by thinking about summertime. By then, the baby will probably sleep through the night and I will feel like a million dollars.

### Getting Moving

As soon as you are able to move, you can begin to help yourself recover by doing exercises. These certainly are not calisthenics, but rather some simple planned movements designed specifically for someone who has just had surgery. These exercises can be very helpful, both physically and emotionally. The nurses may help you get started as the anesthesia wears off. Or, if your husband is present, he can coach you. It is hard to muster the discipline to exercise when you would feel more comfortable holding still, so a coach is almost essential. In this early period, probably any movement will cause some discomfort. However, no activity should continue if it is causing ongoing pain.

Start exercising very slowly, simply taking a deep breath or two. At first, you will find that you cannot take in nearly as much air as you could before the surgery. Then tense and relax each arm and leg separately, as you probably learned to do in your childbirth preparation class. Lying on your back, point your toes away from you, toward the foot of the bed, then up toward the ceiling. Bend one knee at a time, sliding your foot along the bed toward you; then stretch out that leg and repeat with the other. From a position of resting at your side, slowly raise and lower each arm. Then extend your arms so that they are perpendicular to your body, and again raise and lower each arm. Continue to take regular breaths as you exercise. It will be tempting to breathe shallowly, but it is better to breathe deeply. Expand your chest and abdomen somewhat with each inward breath, and contract or pull in the muscles each time you breathe out. This is certainly no time for heroics, but a little extra movement or breathing each time you think of it will be very helpful in preventing lung infections and promoting recovery.

The nurse will ask you to cough or "huff" several times. The purpose of this is to remove secretions that may have settled at the base of your lungs. Coughing also serves to prevent collapse of your lungs, or to re-expand portions that may have collapsed. It is especially important if you have had a general anesthetic. One effective way to do this is not actually coughing in the usual sense, but rather saying "hah" at the same time that you pull in your diaphragm and abdominal muscles sharply. It requires some concentration and will power to perform this exercise, since it may cause pulling on the incision. It may help to place a pillow firmly over the incision while you are huffing. Breathe deeply, then huff several times and breathe deeply again.

> She seemed like such a nice nurse, but after a while she got pushy. Do this, do that. All I said out loud was, "You're kidding!" but I thought to myself that she must have never had an operation or she wouldn't be so firm about all this moving and coughing business.

There is some support for the idea that certain exercises lessen the discomfort caused by gas during the recovery period. The exercises seem more effective if they are begun immediately after the birth. The exercise that is most often recommended is called "abdominal tightening." Take a deep, relaxing breath and let it out. Then take another breath, allowing the abdominal muscles to push gently outward so that your chest and abdomen rise as you expand your lungs. Hold the breath for several seconds. Now slowly release it, pulling in with your abdominal muscles to help squeeze all the remaining air out of your lungs. Make sure you also contract the muscles in the lower abdomen around the incision. Hold for several more seconds. Then take another relaxing breath. Repeat this at least six to eight times a day.

### Going to Your Room

Once your blood pressure, pulse, and rate of breathing are stable and your room is ready, then you (and your IV and catheter) will be moved to a regular maternity floor room. This move can be painful, as you may need to be shifted onto a rolling stretcher and then moved again into your bed. The electric beds usually can be raised almost to the same height as the rolling stretcher, so that it is not too difficult to slide from one to the other. The nurses will help you, but you may feel awkward or scared in spite of their assistance. Some women suffer most just from the loss of decorum, as hospital gowns and peripads slip out of position, particularly with the catheter still in place. It may be easier if the move takes place within the first hour or so after you have received an injection of pain medication.

As part of getting settled into your room, you should have the call bell pinned near your head where you can easily reach it. In addition, find out where the control buttons are for the bed, so that you may begin raising and lowering it by yourself. Every little bit of independence and ability to control your environment helps!

The move from the recovery room to your own room establishes a welcome trend that will continue for days to come—feeling less like a surgical patient and more like a mother. Some women, although they cannot take over very much of the baby's care, feel a strong need to see and hold the baby right away. This may be especially true for women who have had a general anesthetic and did not see the baby at birth.

> I waited so long for the moment when I could hold that precious baby in my arms. And here I was, feeling like half a person. I was determined to get better FAST so I could start being a mother at last.

If you want to see your baby, whether for the first time or to renew your acquaintance, you should ask to have her brought to your room.

For many women, this early recovery period is difficult enough, and they feel grateful for the knowledge that the baby is getting good care in the nursery. Fathers and sometimes even grandparents may spend lots of time with the baby in the nursery and give you full reports of her progress. Occasionally, women feel guilty if they do not want to be with the baby from the start. Yet it is unrealistic to expect yourself to start parenthood with a capital *P* when you are recovering from surgery. There will be plenty of time for you and the baby to become even better acquainted when you are feeling better.

## The First Walk

Sooner or later the moment will come when not just one, but two or three nurses will walk into your room. They are all cheerful and full of determination. You are informed that you are going to take a walk. Before you can protest, they are raising the head of the bed fully and explaining how to inch your way safely toward the side, using the side rails to help you. You will soon find yourself sitting with your feet dangling over the edge of the bed. Then, with support on each side from the nurses, you will slowly stand on your feet and take a few reluctant steps. The practice of getting surgical patients out of bed is called "early ambulation," and its purpose is to improve your circulation and help prevent postoperative complications.

One of the most helpful hints for the first walk is so simple that it seems silly: Don't look at the floor, look forward! You will not be going far, perhaps just to a chair, so fix your eyes on your destination. For some reason, this helps to restore equilibrium and confidence.

Many women are afraid to walk for the first time, either because it hurts or because they worry that their incision may open up. This feeling of being on the verge of coming apart is typical of all surgical patients. In fact, there are many layers of sutures and they are very strong, so the accidental opening of the incision is extremely rare. Despite your fears, it is best to stand up as straight as you can and pull in the lower abdominal muscles gently, to give yourself a feeling of greater support in the incision area.

> I felt so bad at first that I thought I might never walk again. Then they came in and said they were getting me up, and suddenly I didn't want to walk. But I figured they knew best, and besides, I was in no position to argue, so we did it. And I was amazed. I didn't hurt as much as I thought, and I felt better afterward. I also went right to sleep.

If you are still feeling a lot of pain, it may be helpful to have your first walk about forty-five minutes to an hour after you have had some pain medication. However, there is the added problem that the medication makes some people feel dizzy, which certainly will not help you when you are on your feet the first few times.

Some women are very embarrassed when they have a sudden discharge of blood from the vagina on their first few walks. Women who have their babies vaginally have the same problem, and the nurses are used to it. You might not want to wear your slippers the first few times you get on your feet. It is tricky to keep a peripad in position when you are trying to climb out of bed.

There really are good psychological reasons for getting out of bed, in spite of all the attendant problems. Probably the biggest one is that it may help you feel more like a mother and less like an invalid. The other benefit is that you will probably get fresh bed linen while you are out of bed, and this, too, does wonders for your spirits. Even if it seems like torture to get up now, it will be easier the next time, and each walk will be a measure of your progress toward full recovery.

### Feeling a Little Better

After the first walk, other signs of recovery begin to appear. You will be allowed to take something by mouth for the first time. You may start very gradually, perhaps just sucking on a few ice chips. By now, your mouth probably tastes very dry and neglected, so the ice chips are just wonderful! You will graduate to water, and then other clear fluids.

As you begin to move more freely, you will develop the ability to change positions, reach for things, and even sleep with your IV and catheter still in place. The IV needle is taped firmly, hopefully to the opposite hand or arm from the one you use more, and the IV will not be harmed by ordinary movements. If you feel any pain where it is attached, it is a good idea to have it checked. The IV bottles can be attached to a pole on wheels if they are not already, so that you can take them with you when you start getting around on your own.

Some hospitals use "belly binders" for Cesarean mothers.

These are large elastic bandages that are wrapped around the abdomen. Some women feel tremendously relieved to have their abdomen supported in this way, especially when they begin to walk around. Although the initial pressure on the area just above the incision may seem worrisome, the comfort you feel when the binder is applied can be wonderful. The binder usually slips out of position after a while and has to be rewrapped, which the nurses can easily do. Some doctors feel that binders are old-fashioned. If your hospital does not use them, you may ask your doctor's permission to wear a lightweight elastic girdle (probably several sizes larger than any you've ever worn!).

There are special sanitary belts available, designed for Cesarean mothers. The vertical straps are longer so that the straps don't irritate the area of the incision. Many women prefer to avoid belts by using the pads which attach directly to your underpants.

Some hospitals routinely have surgical patients wear long elastic stockings. The nurses can apply them properly and reapply them if they start to sag. They are precautions against circulatory problems, and they probably will feel good. They are usually removed after several days, when you are walking around frequently.

## FEELING MUCH BETTER

### Getting to the Toilet

Many women count the removal of the catheter as a great milestone in recovery. Its removal is quick and painless, but you may wish to do some deep, slow chest breathing in order to remain relaxed while it is being taken out. If it is removed early, then you should ask a nurse to help you get to the bathroom each time until you feel steady on your feet. Even if you feel confident that you can make the trip solo, it is a good precaution to have a nurse standing by the first few times you try it. She will be happy that you decided to take the conservative approach. If you make the mistake of getting into the bathroom without help and then start to feel woozy, there is usually a button to push or a string to pull that will activate the call signal at the nursing station, just as the button at your bedside does.

Some doctors ask that you continue to collect your urine in a cup for another day or two, so that the quantity can be measured. If you are having a little difficulty urinating anyhow, trying to do it into a cup with the nurse standing nearby may be the last straw. Even though you need the nurse's help getting to the bathroom, you may ask her to wait out in the hall or to come back in a few minutes if her presence is making you self-conscious.

Once you can make it to the bathroom, the nurses may also ask you to cleanse your perineal area each time you use the toilet or change your peripad. Your vaginal discharge (lochia) will continue for quite some time, and the cleansing routine is thought to reduce the risk of irritation. Usually it simply involves filling a small plastic squirt bottle with warm water and squirting it over the perineal area as you sit on the toilet. Simple enough, but you may not enjoy the constant reminder of your shaved and unfamiliar-feeling genital area.

### I'm Hungry!

By the second or third day after the baby is born, most Cesarean mothers have graduated to a stage of recovery that is quite comfortable. You are getting about on your own, with short trips down the hall added to your repertoire. The catheter and the IV have been removed. If your doctor is conservative or your intestinal tract slow to recover, you may only be eating broth and Jell-O, while your appetite is at the steak-and-potatoes stage. Even so, real food is not far away, so do not give in to the temptation to cheat. You should avoid carbonated beverages of all kinds, and stick to Sanka until your doctor gives the go-ahead for tea or coffee.

My doctor came in one night at five-thirty and made some crack about me not finishing my Jell-O. So I told him what I thought of the so-called food they were giving me. After he listened to my abdomen with his stethoscope, he said I could have cereal the next morning. Well, when morning came and there was more broth and fruit juice, I felt like crying. I got the nurse to check into it, and she came back with a tray of food, real FOOD!

### Decreasing Medication

Once you can take fluids by mouth, you can also take your medicine that way. The medication is ordered as needed ("PRN"), which means that the staff may assume you are doing fine unless you speak up about feeling uncomfortable. Sooner or later, you will start finding that you don't need medication quite as often and that you don't think about it as much. If you were very uncomfortable at first, then it probably seemed like forever between injections, even though it was actually about four hours. Now, however, you may find that your joy about the baby and your interest in life around you are enough to distract you from the pain. Perhaps your awareness of how sore you are returns late at night when the visitors are gone, the corridors are quiet, and you are too restless to sleep.

> I was higher than a kite. I knew I needed to sleep, but I didn't really want to. I took the sleeping pill and then lay down, but as soon as I started to doze off I also turned over and that woke me up because it hurt a lot. Finally, I called the nurse and told her the problem. She brought a pain pill right away, and then I slept until they brought the baby to nurse at 2:00 A.M.

How do you know if you need the medicine? Trial and error are best. You should certainly ask for the medicine when you are hurting, and do not wait until the pain is so unbearable that you are sure you cannot handle it without medication. This is not an endurance test, and you are not being a baby. On the other hand, after a few days you may not need the medication every time it is offered or every four hours as a matter of course. If medication is offered and you aren't sure if you need it, ask the nurse if she will leave the pills by your bedside. This practice is possible with certain kinds of medication, although it is not legal with other kinds. If the pills are left with you, the nurse will want to know whether you have taken them. She is not checking on your strength of will; hospitals have a legal obligation to record what medicines each patient takes.

Your doctor will be decreasing the strength and frequency of your medication, and he or she will assume that whatever is ordered is making you comfortable unless you let the nurses know otherwise. If you feel you need more medication, be sure to discuss this with your doctor. If you are comfortable without it, you certainly do not have to take it. Your goals for yourself during this period should be to move around freely, enjoy your baby, and rest comfortably and often. These are the keys to the fastest possible recovery.

### Getting Clean

About the third or fourth postpartum day, most women feel distinctly grubby and become concerned about personal appearance. Your hair could certainly use a shampoo. Your sponge baths leave you feeling unbathed. Oh for a shower or bath! The prohibition against baths is common, as doctors are concerned that your cervix has not completely closed. (There is some opening of the cervix toward the end of the pregnancy, even if you have not labored.) The question of whether a shower is medically acceptable is open to considerable debate. Some doctors say that it is not good for either the bandages or the actual area of the incision to get wet. Others say that wet dressings can be replaced and that soap and water are good for the site of the incision. Still others use no bandages at all, preferring simple clear plastic adhesive strips. If you have the good fortune to have a doctor who is inclined to encourage early showers, enjoy!

I started to feel human for the first time. I washed off dried blood and two-day-old perspiration, and I think I also washed away some worries and frustrations. I have been used to starting each day with a shower, and this was even better. I felt like I was starting parenthood, getting clean and fresh and ready to face whatever was wait-

ing out there for me—except that I used to follow my daily shower
by getting dressed and going to work, but this time I followed it
with finding a fresh nightgown and going back to bed for a brief
nap.

### This, Too, Shall Pass

Unfortunately, just when you begin to think that recovery will be
a breeze, a few new variables often arrive on the scene. The first
is the gas pains that most Cesarean mothers feel, and that for a
few are worse than anything they remember about the actual
birth. Your intestines quit functioning when the baby was born,
as they do after any kind of major abdominal surgery. About the
second or third day they begin to work again, and this is when
gas starts moving through the intestinal tract. If you have been
walking around and doing exercises regularly up to this point,
then the gas pains will not be as bad as they otherwise might. If
you experience severe gas pains, they can feel like a serious set-
back.

Even if the gas pains are very bad, this is one case where increasing your intake of medication probably is not helpful, since
the medication can make matters worse in the long run by slowing down your intestinal activity. Walking and other gentle kinds
of exercise are the most tried-and-true therapy. In addition, it
helps to lie on your left side with your legs curled up partway,
then gently knead your abdomen. This is also a good time to use
the breathing exercises you learned in your childbirth preparation
classes, particularly the deep, slow chest breathing. If you continue to be in a great deal of pain, be sure to tell the nurses. A
suppository or a small enema may relieve you, although some
women would rather suffer than endure yet another invasion of
their bodies at this time. A small tube that can be inserted into
the rectum by the nurse carries the same objections, but also may
bring blessed relief.

Once you have begun to pass gas and are eating normally, you
will also finally produce your first bowel movement. This may not
occur for many days after the baby's birth. Drinking lots of fluids

and moving around a lot will help to make the first bowel movement less uncomfortable. There is no reason to worry about how soon it comes, although the fact that the nurses keep asking if you have moved your bowels yet may make you more nervous than is warranted.

### Breast Discomfort

The other new source of discomfort occurs when your milk comes in. Your breasts will start to feel tender and begin to swell. Soon they are engorged and the slightest touch may hurt. If you are breast-feeding, this will happen a little sooner because of the stimulation to your nipples. The quantity of milk will eventually even out, and in the meantime the best relief for you will be to let the baby nurse.

If your baby is being bottle-fed, the matter becomes a little more complicated. There is an injection that may be given to women in order to help dry up their milk. It is certainly not helpful in every case, and its use is decreasing as concern about its effectiveness and its side effects increases. You may find yourself just hoping that this part of your adjustment will be over soon. The application of heat helps some women, while ice packs help others. Some hospitals still bind women's breasts, although this seems not to help a great deal, and may increase the risk of infection. A good supportive bra is a must, and nursing pads may be used to prevent milk from leaking and staining your nightgown. (Nursing pads are usually available from the nurses.) You may cut back on your fluid intake a very small amount. Anything more will have a negative effect on your recovery from surgery. Your breasts will probably start returning to their prepregnant state by the time you are ready to leave the hospital, although the nipples may feel tender and easily stimulated for several weeks.

### Comfort Measures

Some hospitals provide gowns that are both pretty and comfortable. In fact, they may have some advantages that you have not thought of. For one thing, the supply is endless, meaning that you can get into something fresh each morning and again before you go to bed at night, or even more often if you wish. Along with fresh bed linen, this can be very soothing. In addition, the gowns are probably made of cotton, which is better for you because it absorbs perspiration and does not contribute to your slipping and sliding all around your bed. As a postsurgical and postpartum patient, you may have periods of suddenly becoming very sweaty. This is a normal part of your recovery, but hard on the wardrobe. A further advantage is that they open easily. There are obstetrical hospital gowns designed especially for nursing mothers. But with a slight risk of looking undignified, any hospital gown can be turned so the open part is in front. If you wish to begin wearing your own clothes, a new loose robe or caftan can do a lot for your morale.

### The Blues
Most mothers experience periods of feeling very emotional during some part of their hospital stay, and often these feelings continue to crop up after you go home. Although this phenomenon has been tagged "the blues," it may not feel that way to you when it happens. Sometimes it is just a matter of being very emotional, crying at the slightest provocation. Your husband brings you a rose, and suddenly you are sobbing, all the while saying how beautiful it is and how happy you are. In some cases, though, the tears are associated with real disappointments or frustrations. Since everyone expects you to have some blue periods, you may have the infuriating experience of being told "You'll feel better after a while" instead of having your complaints dealt with on their merits.

### Making Friends
As you begin to feel better, you also begin wanting to re-expand the borders of the world you live in. You can start by getting to know other mothers on the floor. Perhaps the nurses will introduce you to another Cesarean mother. If she has just had her Cesarean the day before, it will be very encouraging for her to see

you on your fourth or fifth postpartum day looking very spry. If her recovery is at a similar stage to yours, it will be fun for you simply to exchange birth stories and admire each other's baby. Sometimes a nurse may have passed on a tip on how to be more comfortable to another mother but forgotten to share it with you. Although you may not feel like you have a lot to give right now, experience has shown that Cesarean mothers often can offer support to each other that is invaluable.

### Taking Out the Stitches

Somewhere around the fifth day of your hospital stay, or perhaps a little later, your stitches or clamps will be removed. This is a nerve-wracking time for most women. You have little support from your abdominal muscles, so that part of your body feels untrustworthy, somehow. In addition, you feel very vulnerable after surgery, so the prospect of someone tampering with your body once more may seem really unpleasant. And many women are just scared that the removal of the stitches or the clamps will plunge them back into pain.

The actual event of having the stitches taken out is nothing like the fears many women have about it. The pain is no more than a slight sting. Some women feel nothing at all. The incision is healing well at this point and the danger of rupture is almost nil. Once the stitches have been removed, a new dressing (bandages) may be applied, or simple transparent strips with an adhesive back may be used. If you do get a new dressing, you may be sent home with it and asked to come to the doctor's office in a few days to have it removed.

While the site of the incision is still completely uncovered, it is a good idea to ask for a mirror to see what the area looks like. There will be the incision itself, perhaps still quite darkened where dried blood remains, and dark red in the other parts. There may be areas that look bruised around the incision. And your stretch marks, if you had any, will still be there. Although this is not a lovely sight, it is probably not as bad as you imagined either. And it is helpful for you to look at it now, so that you do not go home and stand in front of the mirror for the first time wondering if that is the way it is supposed to look.

## UNDERSTANDING YOUR BIRTH EXPERIENCE

As you begin to feel better, you also have more resources to take stock of what happened. Perhaps the birth was everything you hoped for. For most couples, even those who had time to plan their Cesarean in advance, there are some things that come as a surprise or that were not what they hoped for.

> My doctor and I agreed on a spinal. Well, it all went smoothly, Michael was born and they let Jim in and we were just so happy! But then I started to feel uncomfortable while they were stitching me up. That's all I remember, because the anesthesiologist put me to sleep right then. I don't remember much of that day the baby was born, and I am just furious! I was pretty smug, thinking we had it all planned this time, and then this had to happen. When I am feeling better, I intend to give that guy a piece of my mind.

As you begin to think about your birth experience, particularly if it was an unplanned Cesarean, you will have many questions. It is important to get your questions answered as thoroughly as possible. Hopefully, your husband can be present for one or more meetings with your doctor in which you go over what happened, why it happened, and what you may expect in the weeks to come. The advantages to your being together for your talk with the doctor are that there is a lot of information to absorb, and you probably will recall it more easily as a couple. In addition, your husband may well have some questions or concerns that never occurred to you. Finally, coping with major surgery is not easy. If neither of you has had surgery before, you have no idea what you may realistically expect. Although the surgery happened to you, much of the responsibility for helping you recover will be on your husband's shoulders, so each of you has a need for information and support as you prepare for the weeks to come.

Research suggests that Cesarean mothers who receive a forty-five-minute session of postpartum teaching by a trained nurse feel better about their birth experience and about their recovery than women who are not given this information. The principle involved here is very simple: You absorb and adjust best to that which you understand. Most women know basically why their Cesarean was done, but many express a need to know much more. Why did I labor so long? Did I do anything that contributed to having a Cesarean? So many questions occur sometimes that it is good to write them down and keep a list. Some hospitals have added classes about Cesarean birth to the usual roster of postpartum classes on bathing and breast-feeding. There are excellent visual aids available now, which meet the normal desire of many women to see a Cesarean birth so that they can further know what happened to them.

> Since they had to put me to sleep, it was like it didn't happen. The doctor went over it all and gave me something to read, but it still seemed like something that happened to someone else. I would look at the baby and remember being pregnant, and there was nothing to help me get from pregnancy to baby in my mind. When I finally saw a movie showing a Cesarean, I cried. I don't know why. It was the relief, I guess, of finally knowing how my baby got here.

## YOUR CHILDREN AT HOME

If you have older children at home who are not permitted to visit, you may feel yourself pulled in several different directions all at once. You feel very limited in what you can do, so the idea of remaining in the hospital as long as your doctor advises seems appealing. The time when you have to take on much more responsibility will come soon enough! Yet you miss your older child terribly, and may feel guilty about the long separation as well. It would be so reassuring to both of you if you could cuddle your older child and let him know that you haven't abandoned him.

Now many hospitals are allowing children to visit mothers (officially called "sibling visitation," although the important person being visited from the child's standpoint is Mother!). This has proved to be a very popular change in hospital practices, and it probably benefits Cesarean mothers most of all, since their hospital stay is usually about twice as long as that of women who deliver vaginally. The child who can see for himself or herself that mother is alive and (reasonably) well will feel very reassured. Sometimes children (and mothers!) cry at the end of the visit, leaving you to worry whether no visit at all would have been better than one that ended so painfully. Yet in the end, sibling visitation has been greeted wih tremendous enthusiasm by parents and children wherever it has been implemented.

If visitation is not allowed, there are certainly other ways that you can keep in touch with your children. If you have or can borrow an instant camera, family members can bring pictures back and forth from home to hospital and vice versa. If your children are old enough to appreciate notes or a phone call, these are ideal ways to communicate. Your messages should be short, and you can take your cues from your child as to what his concerns are. He may be more interested in telling you about the frog he caught than he is in hearing about his new baby brother or sister. Keep in mind that the baby is still a very abstract concept to the older child, while the separation from you and the day-to-day events of his life have much more reality.

Some mothers have put a small tape recorder to good use at this time. You can make short tapes, just chatting or perhaps reading favorite stories or singing songs your older child enjoys. These have the advantage of being repeatable, and they don't leave you wondering what your toddler is thinking while he nods and smiles into the phone. An older child of four or more may wish to make a tape to send back to you. If your children are close in age, you may find that your not-much-older child at home finds the tape confusing, since he cannot understand the presence of Mommy's voice when she is absent.

## GOING HOME

Once you are given your doctor's permission to leave the hospital, you may be flooded with excitement, anticipation, and concern all at once. You probably didn't realize how much you brought with you until you tried to pack it all to go home. And you have acquired some cards, perhaps some flowers, along with a collection of personal aids such as nursing pads, hand cream, etc. Suddenly, leaving the hospital seems like a major production! It helps if you pack a little at a time, resting as you go. Perhaps your partner can arrive early and help you prepare to leave. A paper bag or two will accommodate the overflow. It also helps to be realistic in your plans, so the fact that you don't make it home until after lunchtime does not come as an unpleasant surprise.

If this is the first time you have dressed in your own clothes, you may have a shock in store for you. It is really unlikely that you will be able to wear anything but maternity clothes, unless you have a wrap-around skirt to press into service. Even if you have already lost most of the weight you gained in pregnancy, your abdominal muscles are still stretched out. In addition, close-fitting clothing may put pressure on your scar, creating some discomfort. Although it may not help your morale, you should dress for comfort, not for style.

Some women find that leaving the hospital is a very emotional time. Saying good-bye to the nurses or packing up the "nest" that you have made for yourself in your hospital room may bring tears to your eyes. Or you may be feeling quite calm. Most hospitals require that you ride to the door in a wheelchair and some insist that a nurse carry the baby. What a procession: You in the wheelchair, perhaps holding the baby; your husband holding your suitcase in one hand and a bouquet of flowers in the other; and an extra bag of things tucked into the wheelchair with you. The nurse who is pushing you is accustomed to these things, although you may feel like you are in a parade.

Getting into the car can be a major production, too. The baby should be tucked into his infant seat, a procedure you may find quite unwieldy at first. If you have not been allowed to see your older child, a reunion will occur at last. Your older child may hang back shyly or want to sit on your lap immediately. He may want to look over the new family member, but many children only give the baby a short glance. Then all the suitcases, bags, etc., have to find their place in the car.

Joey always used to ride in back because I read that it was safer. When we left the hospital to bring the baby home, Joey suddenly decided that his place was in front. He made quite a fuss about it. Thank goodness Joe took over. He calmed Joey down and switched the car seats around so that the baby was in back and Joey in front between us. I decided it was better that way. Peace and quiet, plus I really didn't want to just shove the baby down Joey's throat. There would be plenty of times soon when he would be the one having to accommodate to the baby.

As they leave the hospital, many women feel a sense of strangeness. If the baby was born at a time of rapid change in the season, you may be startled to learn that the buds have opened, or the fall leaves have begun to change color. Sometimes it is just an adjustment to the way the outdoors looks and feels after the long period of being so enclosed. Your comfort in the car may be increased if your husband reassures you that he will be at his most cautious while driving. It also helps to have a small pillow to place over your incision, especially if you are holding the baby or if you have the good habit of wearing your seatbelt.

And then, at last, you are on your way home.

# NINE

# You and the New Baby at Home

You are finally home. Even though you looked forward to this day, you may feel a mixture of elation and dread. This baby is totally yours now. But do you really know how to take care of a baby? You will spend the night in your own bed. But will you have the strength to leave it and get through the next day? The mood swings that are common for all parents may be even more intense when you have a Cesarean delivery.

I was so excited to be going home. My husband and I dressed the baby in the outfit her grandmother had brought the day before. The nurses smiled and waved as they wished us luck. We drove about two miles and the baby began to cry. She cried the rest of the way home and for about fifteen minutes after that. The short trip just exhausted me. I wished someone from the nursery would come and help. Maybe the baby was happier in the hospital. I knew right then I wished I were safe in my hospital bed.

Some couples expect parenthood to be a life of never-ending bliss. If their own lives don't immediately work out that way, they may feel that it is because they are doing something wrong.

Whether this is their first child or they are old hands at parenting, a new infant will change family routines and relationships. It may seem that everything is in an uproar for a while.

There are so many good things that will happen during the first weeks and months with your baby—in fact, for the rest of your life now that you are a parent. You will know when these occur and how to enjoy them! This chapter focuses on those times that may not be all that pleasant—the problems that can occur in any family. Thankfully, you won't encounter every difficulty we mention (at least not all at once). It takes time and flexibility to incorporate a new person into your family. After a Cesarean, you are adjusting to a baby and major surgery. You may have to repeat this phrase to yourself over and over during the next few weeks!

## TAKING CARE OF YOURSELF

Becoming a mother is a major step for any woman. When you have had a Cesarean delivery, you may be especially aware that maintaining a balance between your needs and those of the rest of your newly-expanded family can take a certain amount of juggling on your part.

### Getting Enough Rest
After a Cesarean delivery, your biggest need is enough rest. One of the best things you can do for yourself is to make sure you will have help when you come home from the hospital. Perhaps your husband can take a week or two of vacation time. Although this usually gives the whole family more time together for these first exciting days, it may not be the entire answer to your need for rest. Your husband is tired, too. After all, both of you have just been through a pretty exhausting experience. Also, even if you have been sharing household jobs before your baby's birth, it will be difficult for him to continue doing his share in addition to

yours while helping with the baby and giving you the special care you need.

Your mother, mother-in-law, sister, or other family member can sometimes spend a week or ten days with you. This works very well for some women, but others suspect that having a relative in their home for this length of time would do more harm than good. You may be faced with deciding if the help they can give you is more important than the wear and tear on your nerves. If your mother is the type who will give constant advice on the one and only route to perfect parenting, you might want to explore other avenues of help. Families who can afford it often find that a temporary housekeeper is the best answer. She is comfortable entering other people's homes and taking over household routines. If you are the kind of woman who finds it hard to ask for help, you may feel more comfortable with someone you have employed to assist you. No matter what kind of assistance you arrange for, make sure you make use of it once you are home. Sometimes it is very difficult to ask someone else to fold the laundry or clean your bathroom. You may find that you are doing these things while your helper holds the baby or fixes gourmet meals.

You probably have never had to be this dependent on other people. If you are unprepared for the periods of overwhelming fatigue that can follow a Cesarean birth, you may feel guilty about the slowness of your recovery. Women sometimes feel self-indulgent or weak when they take frequent naps. Anyone who has had surgery feels tired during the recovery period. Your fatigue is worse, since you are no doubt getting up a few times each night to feed your baby. Resting may take a great effort on your part. You don't want to feel so tired. But be strong. Take a nap.

I would get into bed and then I would start remembering all the things that needed to be done. I would really try to get to sleep but I just couldn't even though I was so tired. I would see piles of laundry, dirty dishes, and unpaid bills. Then I would hear the baby cry and even though my sister had said she would take care of him, I would crawl out of bed because I felt it was my DUTY to be with my baby.

Even though your energy seemed to be returning when you had help, you may find that you are really tired again once the help is gone. For some women the first few days alone, after housekeeper or relative has left and husband has returned to work, are especially difficult. Readjusting their expectations about what they can do during any one day is hard for many women. Let the laundry pile up, ask someone else to make the phone calls you were going to do for your parenting group, and ignore the files you were going to get in order during your leave from work. There are some women who can resume their full life shortly after their baby is born, but many need six weeks or more (six months to a year isn't all that unusual) before they are ready to take on the world again. If neighbors or friends ask what they can do to help, be honest and let them aid you. A casserole for dinner or a friend who can come to spend some time with you, especially during the afternoon, can make life a lot easier. If your husband can come home a half hour earlier than usual for a while, this may be helpful.

### Visitors

One decision almost all couples must make is how to share the joy of their new baby with the world without becoming overtired and exposed to more advice, germs, and company than they can possibly cope with. At times when you don't want to see visitors, you may have to be more assertive than you have ever been in your life, or at least allow your husband or helper to be assertive for you. Try to get the word out to friends and relatives that you would love to see them at a specific time during the day. For instance, if your most lively time is around one o'clock in the afternoon, that would be a good time to see company. Also, during these first few weeks at home, it is a good idea to keep any visit fairly short. Don't feel you have to entertain or provide refreshments to people who drop in. You just can't do that right now. If you are really tired, allow whoever is there to help you to give your regrets to your callers, and let them know you will phone them (if this appeals to you), and assure them that they will see the baby soon. Sometimes not seeing friends who call takes a great deal of strength on your part.

If you have a toddler or even a four-, five-, or six-year-old at home and you know there will be many gifts brought to the house for the new baby, keep a supply of small "treasures" to share with your older child in case visitors forget to bring something for both children. Older children have problems adjusting to new babies as it is. Watching their younger sibling being showered with gifts while they feel ignored may aggravate any hostile feelings they have. You will not be spoiling your older child during this short time of change in your lives.

### As Your Body Changes

Even if you were feeling quite comfortable in the hospital with little or no medication, it is usually a good idea to have a prescription to take home with you when you are discharged. Often your doctor will offer to do this. If he or she doesn't, feel free to request it. Your activity level increases considerably once you are home. The hospital was arranged so you had to travel the minimum amount of distance among baby, bed, and bathroom. Most homes require a lot more walking to reach those same goals. Even if you feel you are resting a great deal of the time, there are many more demands on you at home than there were in the hospital. Also, some women just feel pain longer than others. You may find that you never need to take a pill after you are home, or you may need one once or twice during your first few days. For some women, just knowing it's available is comfort enough.

Sometimes, when women have had a great deal of soreness following a Cesarean delivery, they are especially hesitant to stop taking medication for fear the pain will come rushing back. This worry is not uncommon. Many find it helpful gradually to increase the interval between pills, rather than stopping them altogether. It is not likely that you will become addicted to the medication during this short time.

Another concern is the effect of the pills on the baby when breast-feeding. All medication does reach the baby in some amount. If you are nursing, discuss the possible effects of the particular medication with your doctor. (See Chapter Seven for complete discussion of breast-feeding after a Cesarean.)

Your incision, which was once very painful, gradually begins to feel sore and tender. This can happen either a few days or up to a week or so after birth. During this time you will be very aware that any activity has an effect on your lower abdomen. For at least several weeks after that you may be conscious of the incision but it is not really sore or uncomfortable. After a time, it will begin to itch. (Some women experience itching from the first postpartum day on.) Although itching means healing is taking place, realizing this may not give you much comfort while it is going on. The itching certainly isn't constant, but it does come and go with varying degrees of intensity and sometimes at most inappropriate times. Don't be surprised if intermittent itching recurs for a few months after your baby is born.

> It seemed that whenever I went out my incision would begin to itch. It happened in the grocery store and in my doctor's office. The worst time was one night in a theater lobby. There we stood with another couple a few months after our daughter was born and all I could think was that I wished it were acceptable to scratch in public in our society. I became very adept at surreptitiously moving my arm across my lower abdomen.

As your incision heals, it goes through changes in appearance. At first it looks quite large and reddish-purple. There may also be areas of bruised skin around the incision. As the color begins to fade, the scar tends to become raised and bumpy in places. Usually within a few months, the scar smoothes out and becomes a thin white line. It really does become virtually unnoticeable with time, especially if you had a "bikini" incision which falls below your pubic hairline.

Most women who have Cesarean deliveries have no problems with incision infections. However, if your incision gets red or puffy, or feels wet to you or becomes increasingly more tender, you should get in touch with your doctor. In fact, if you are really concerned but have none of these symptoms, it is always best to go ahead and call the doctor so your mind will be put at rest.

Almost all women experience some twinges and occasional pain around the incision during the first weeks, and these symptoms make many women wonder if something is going wrong. Minor pain can occur if you are getting adequate rest, but it is more likely to happen if you have been overdoing it. Then your body may be trying to tell you that you are just doing too much.

By the time you come home from the hospital, your vaginal discharge has probably become a thin, brownish-red flow which will eventually become brownish-yellow. This discharge is called lochia and will likely go on for another two to six weeks. You will probably be most comfortable if you continue to use sanitary napkins that attach directly to your underwear rather than using a belt. Also, many doctors prefer that you do not use tampons until after your six-week visit so they can be sure that your reproductive organs have returned to normal.

If you are not breast-feeding, your first spontaneous menstruation will occur about six weeks after you deliver. For nursing mothers, it may not occur until you begin giving your baby solid foods, or sometimes until your baby is almost totally weaned. In either case, your first period may not seem "normal" to you. Often the flow is much heavier or much lighter than what you experienced before you became pregnant. Some women report that the area around the incision becomes unusually tender each month just before and during menstruation. This may happen for only a few months, or for much longer.

### Eating Well

It's always important to eat well, but during the time you are recovering from a Cesarean birth (remember—baby *and* surgery) it is especially so. Your body is recuperating from the shock of the operation as well as adjusting to the new routines of parenting. You need the energy you get from well-balanced meals as you rebuild your strength and take care of your baby. During this time it is also important to drink plenty of fluids, especially if you are nursing your baby.

Good fluid intake and balanced meals also help make moving

your bowels easier. Even after you return home, the act of moving your stools may be uncomfortable, since it puts pressure on your incision. Fruits, vegetables, and roughage in your diet help keep your bowels as soft as possible. If you have a great deal of difficulty you should talk to your doctor about a stool softener.

When you are recovering from a Cesarean delivery, fixing well-balanced meals is often one of the last things you worry about. It may be a great temptation to eat a lot of snacks rather than prepare a full meal. This will work as long as you eat salads or fruit and steer away from a steady diet of sweets and potato chips. If you find you are serving your entire family convenience foods for a short time after the baby is born, you are certainly doing no irreparable harm. Some packaged foods and "fast food" restaurants are better for you than others. If you are going to eat out, find a restaurant with a salad bar. At home, frozen pizzas "with everything," packaged precooked chicken or fish, granola bars, yogurt, and pudding mixes that you add your own milk to are sound choices. Your best bet is to read the package labels in the grocery store, so you know what you are buying.

### Restrictions on Activities

When you leave the hospital, your doctor may put certain limitations on your activities. Some doctors present women with a long list of do's and don'ts. Some tell you to do whatever you are comfortable doing. These last assume you will know when you are becoming overtired and further assume you will have the sense to stop. If your doctor is the trusting type, you may have to exert a lot of self-control during your first weeks at home.

STAIRS Many times your doctor will suggest that you limit your trips up or down the stairs. The major reason is that climbing stairs is physically exhausting, not that you would cause any damage to your incision. If there are stairs that must be negotiated in your house, make sure you plan rest times between trips. It is best to arrange to spend most of your time on one floor or the other. You can assemble most of what you and your baby need (diapers, bottles—if you are using them, light snacks for you and any older children) in one place and create a "nest" where you can spend most of your time. You may still have to ask someone else to carry the laundry up and down, or even bring you the morning paper. It's better to swallow your pride and ask than to be a martyr and do without. And it is definitely better to ask someone to do these things than to make unnecessary trips yourself.

DRIVING   Some doctors do not want you to drive until after your six-week checkup. Women sometimes feel weak, dizzy, or disoriented their first few times driving after delivery. Once you have been given a go-ahead, you might want to make your first few trips relatively short. Another good policy is to take your first few drives by yourself. Leave your baby at home until you feel really secure behind the wheel again. It is very difficult to concentrate on traffic when you are alone in the car with a crying baby.

TUB BATHS   In the past, doctors used to suggest that women not take a tub bath for the first few weeks after delivery. Most now agree that this is entirely permissible, and if you feel like taking a bath it will very likely do you a world of good. Many women really enjoy a bath, finding it one of the best ways for them to relax. If you are one of these women, just be careful. It is a good idea to take a bath when there is someone around to help you into and out of the tub. Also, only partially filling the tub makes it easier to get in and out. Although the doctor says you may take a bath, you still might want to take showers for a while, since this involves less bending and stretching for you.

LIFTING   You may be told not to lift anything heavier than your baby for the first few weeks. Although you can usually find ways to cope with this limitation—someone else can lift the diaper pail or carry out the trash—you may have problems if you have a younger child at home. You will find some suggestions on handling this later in this chapter.

## Your Six-week Checkup

You will be asked to schedule an appointment with your obstetrician for about six weeks after your delivery. Your doctor will want to make sure your healing has continued and that your reproductive organs have returned to normal.

This visit is a good time to ask any questions that have come up since you left the hospital. It is always a good idea to keep lists as the questions occur to you. Your doctor will probably want to discuss some method of birth control with you. It is best to have researched available methods so you are fairly certain about which you would prefer to use. (Please see bibliography.)

Often women think of this visit as an end to the pregnancy. They somehow expect that with this visit everything, both physically and emotionally, should be resolved. When they leave the doctor's office, still tired, still faced with night feedings and lack of sleep, or still bothered by unresolved feelings about the Cesarean, they may feel cut off from any support system. This six-week checkup is necessary to monitor how your body is doing after the delivery. If you can avoid it, don't invest too much in it emotionally. You are now a parent and will remain so forever. Unfortunately, the difficulties and adjustments in your life will not go away because you have seen the doctor. If you are feeling let down or low, your doctor will not be surprised if you mention it. Perhaps he or she can make some recommendations to help you through this time. Often your doctor will suggest that you become involved with a group of new mothers. There are enormous benefits in sharing the joys and frustrations of these first few months as a mother. It is especially good if you can locate a group of mothers who have had Cesarean deliveries, too.

## Getting Back in Shape

Sometime during these weeks you will probably feel an overwhelming urge to begin getting your body back into shape. Usually you lose between ten and fourteen pounds when your baby is born, a combination of the weight of your baby, the placenta, and the amniotic fluid. Most women lose a few additional pounds during their first week or two postpartum. After that, shedding excess pounds and regaining muscle tone become much harder.

You can continue the stretching and tightening exercises you began in the hospital until you visit your doctor for your postpartum checkup. At this time you can talk over a sensible diet and a long-range exercise program. Resist the temptation to try a "crash diet" even though you may find it enticing to think of pounds "melting away overnight." These diets can be difficult on your system any time, and they may be particularly draining right now. Also, if you are nursing your baby, it is essential that you eat well-balanced meals and drink plenty of fluids. This doesn't mean that you should use your breast-feeding as an excuse for retaining pounds you don't need. You can still watch what you eat and eliminate foods that are filled with empty calories (chocolate cake and pecan pie immediately come to mind). Some women find that they eat more, and especially more foods high in sugar, when they are feeling low. It may be especially hard under these circumstances to lose weight until your emotions are in better balance.

It may be easier for you to begin a diet than to begin an exercise program. There are some excellent programs specificially designed for women who have recently given birth that any woman —super athletic to abnormally clumsy—can do right in her living room. (Please see bibliography.) However, many women find that their bodies really begin to return to shape only when they resume their prepregnancy activities. If you enjoyed jogging, riding a bike, or playing tennis before your baby was born, you will probably look forward to doing these things again. Obviously, they will be more difficult to fit into your schedule now than they were before your baby was born. You may have to find someone to care for your baby while you care for your body. You will also be tired a lot of the time and may just not feel the same amount of zest for strenuous physical activity once you reach the tennis courts. If you led a fairly sedentary life before you became a parent, you should proceed rather carefully now. If you want to begin an exercise program, try building up slowly, so that your enthusiasm and your energy won't suffer early deaths.

One day after my baby was born, I saw these jogging shoes and bought them. I drove home with visions of the Boston Marathon dancing before me. I made it around the block, huffing and puffing all the way. The next day my body was so sore I could barely move.

### As Time Goes On

Life as a Cesarean mother becomes easier. Your strength comes back. You establish routines for taking care of your baby and yourself. None of these happens overnight. In fact, they may be so gradual that it will not occur to you until months afterward that you once again have enough energy to get through the entire day without a nap, or that the thought of someone coming to visit no longer throws you into partial panic.

As soon as you feel up to it, you should arrange times when you can be "off duty" and get out of the house for a bit. You need time just for yourself. A trip to the library, a park, or doing some necessary errands can give you a chance to recoup. You are still a person with needs of your own. Devoting every waking (and semiwaking) moment to the task of motherhood is comfortable for some women. However, many others need time to themselves. Giving yourself time off can make mothering much more enjoyable on your return.

One night, about two months after the baby was born, I had this startling revelation as I was sitting there reading a book. The thing that swept over me was that I had been reading for almost a whole hour without once thinking about motherhood with a capital *M*. I was just really enjoying myself knowing that the baby was asleep and my brain was still capable of comprehending something other than Dr. Spock.

## TAKING CARE OF YOUR BABY

There are many skills involved in taking care of a baby. Changing diapers, giving a bath, and rocking a baby may all take time and practice. It would be much easier if there were a button a man or woman could push when a baby was born. Then everyone would automatically feel comfortable caring for their baby. Since this magic button doesn't exist, new parents must rely to a great extent on trial and error. The more you can do to help one another as you learn to care for this baby, the easier life will be.

## Physical Care

Babies seem to accumulate a lot of possessions in a short time. In no time you are negotiating around a crib, changing table, stroller, high chair, swing, baby bathtub, infant seat, and various other pieces of baby equipment. It is fun to buy things for a new baby and a great temptation for many new parents. The rest of the family still needs space in which to live, however, and you should maintain some sense of balance. Some equipment is especially useful to Cesarean parents. A portable crib or bassinet that rolls from room to room with you can be very helpful. You can take the baby wherever you go and save many trips. Some type of changing table that helps you avoid bending while dressing or changing the baby is a good idea, too. Many women find the baby carriers that hang in front (an extremely good one is Huggle Bunny)[1] and can safely support a young infant useful. You can keep your baby with you and at the same time keep your arms free to do other things. Plastic infant seats are a help, too, since you can safely sit the baby next to you while you work or get a bath ready. (Just make sure you buckle the baby in!) Often you can borrow some of these things from friends whose children have outgrown them. Although some new parents hesitate to use "hand-me-downs" for their first baby, it really makes a great deal of sense.

The more you can do to simplify caring for your baby after a Cesarean delivery, the better. You might want to have your baby

[1] Huggle Bunny is made by La Leche and is a dependable, inexpensive baby carrier. You can contact your local La Leche chapter and see if they have any on hand, or write to: Huggle Bunny, 917 Hendricks Dr., Monroe, MI. 48161.

sleep in the same room with you for a time after you come home. You won't have to travel very far for those middle-of-the-night feedings. You also won't have to make a trip down the hall each time the baby sighs, gurgles, or cries for a minute. It's a lot easier if you just have to roll over and take a peek. Some parents elect to have the baby sleep in their bed with them. Some bring the baby to bed for a late-night feeding, and somehow the baby is never returned to his own quarters. Other parents never take their baby into their bed. Although many "experts" have strong feelings about the risks or benefits of any one system, the best way is really whatever works best for you.

If there is any way for you to make arrangements to use a diaper service or disposable diapers after a Cesarean birth, do so. Although both may be expensive, either will save time and energy that you will need for other things. Often friends or relatives ask what you would like as a gift. You might suggest that they chip in together for a few months of diaper service or a case of disposable diapers. If you have been told not to lift anything after your Cesarean, it may be essential that you find an alternative to washing diapers yourself. There are few things heavier than a pailful of soaking diapers.

### Emotional Care

There will be moments when taking care of your baby gives you more pleasure than anything you have ever done. At other times you will feel like screaming in frustration because nothing you do seems to make this baby happy. There are few absolutes involved in caring for a young baby. The things you do one day that bring smiles and gurgles may bring nothing but cries of indignation the next day. It is hard when you are tired and sore to love your baby twenty-four hours a day. It is not always pleasant to get up in the middle of the night to feed your baby. And yet there are times when sitting alone with your child at two o'clock in the morning is the most peaceful, wonderful thing you could think of doing. Taking care of a baby is a lot like an unending roller-coaster ride. You have ups and downs, but you never get off the ride.

It can take some time to get "tuned in" to your baby. "Tuned in" refers to the messages your baby gives to you concerning her needs. Babies cry to let you know a number of things. They may be hungry, wet, uncomfortable, tired, or lonely. Usually, after a while, you can interpret what they need, although it may take some detective work on your part. Sometimes babies just need to cry. How you decide to handle this is a very individual matter. Some parents prefer to continue holding their infant to provide physical contact during this time. Some choose to give their baby time to cry it out on her own. This is just one of the many times that you will have to experiment to discover which approach makes you more comfortable. The other point to be made is that it takes time to develop the expertise to distinguish this new language your baby uses. You will have to allow yourself time to understand what you are being "told," just as it sometimes takes a while truly to understand what a new acquaintance is saying to you.

Someday I will write a book called *My Most Frustrating Moments as a Mother*. The first chapter will be about the night our son cried for two hours straight right as we were ready to go to bed. We went through our usual bag of tricks. I fed him. I walked him. Bill rocked him. We both tried lullabies. Nothing was working. Bill finally decided the baby had colic. Remembering something his mother had told him God only knows when, he went in search of a hot water bottle. There he was combing the streets at 11:00 P.M. for an all-night drugstore while I was alone with this extremely unhappy baby.

### Are You Really Alone?

When families were closer, it was fairly easy to call your mother or an older sister with questions about diaper rash or a new tooth. Now that many new parents live hundreds or thousands of miles from their nearest relative, this kind of support is not always available. Sometimes, too, you have read so much about parenting or taken your duties so seriously that you are embarrassed asking someone to help you through one of these minor crises. If the baby has a crying spell, you may think you have done something to cause it. This just isn't true. Others have been through this before and you can benefit from their experience.

Friends with young children can be especially helpful while you are learning to care for your baby. Even if your approaches to parenthood are different, there are always common concerns and ways of solving problems that can be helpful. Just knowing someone else's baby was up for three nights in a row, too, can take some of the edge off the exhaustion and exasperation you might be feeling. A friend who has time to talk, even if only by phone, can be a real boost. For many mothers the time between 3:00 P.M. and 6:00 P.M. seems to stretch out forever. Knowing that there is someone you can turn to during this time can become something you look forward to each day.

One day my friend Beverly and I were sitting watching our babies play. We were talking about books, plants, and just "things." Bev sighed long and hard and said something about motherhood being hard. I said I understood. All of a sudden I heard myself telling her that sometimes I just wanted to walk out and close the door. I had the fantasy of going to Chicago and becoming a waitress while waiting for my big break in television. She absolutely grinned from ear to ear. She said that her fantasy was to pack up and become a beach bum in Malibu.

Some childbirth preparation groups now sponsor classes or discussion groups for new parents. Groups often mix practical hints on caring for your baby with an opportunity to share your concerns with other new parents. In some areas, it is possible to arrange for a public health nurse to visit after you come home from the hospital. Some areas routinely send a nurse to visit all Cesarean mothers. This can be very reassuring, as the nurse can answer a lot of questions about your baby as well as any you might have about your own recovery.

### A Big Responsibility
Things that didn't cause you much worry in the hospital can suddenly seem very frightening when you are alone with your infant. A cough, a sneeze, or a crying spell can throw parents into a

minor frenzy. Most parents have read or heard about childhood diseases, and in the back of their minds is the fear that they will miss a sign of impending illness. Even worse, they fear they may actually do something to make their child ill.

> I think that I spent the first month of life with my baby clutching Dr. Spock in one hand. A pimple meant the beginning of chicken pox. A burp meant intestinal problems, and a sneeze was sure to lead directly to pneumonia. I knew more about the exotic illnesses of childhood than anyone needed to know. I was ready to call my pediatrician ten times a day and twenty times each night.

Babies do get sick. They get colds, ear infections, and a variety of other ailments. It can be hard to take care of a sick infant. Usually it is a scary, insecure time for both parents. If you are still recovering from your Cesarean, the added demands on your time and energy may be very difficult.

### Finding a Pediatrician

Your pediatrician will be very important to your whole family for a number of years, so the effort it takes to find one who is supportive is well worth it. It is more accepted now for parents to set up interviews with pediatricians even before the baby is born. This may take time and entail some expense on your part, but you can learn a lot about an individual doctor's ability to communicate (an essential skill for any pediatrician). During this interview you might want to discuss some general areas with the doctor such as his or her views on feeding during the first year and how he or she manages common childhood illnesses.

In addition to the pediatrician, you should feel comfortable with the staff in his or her office. Many times your phone call will be handled by the receptionist or a nurse. Often, too, pediatricians employ nurse practitioners who respond to phone inquiries and may do most well baby checkups. This appeals to some families, since they feel a nurse practitioner may have more time to answer routine questions about their baby. Other parents prefer to be seen by the doctor whether their baby is sick or in for just a checkup.

Since many times you will feel in the greatest need of medical advice late at night or on a weekend, you may wish to check on how local pediatricians handle after-hours calls. Some pediatricians join together to provide services to patients through a clinic staffed on a rotating basis during this time. Although you won't always speak to your own doctor, this does provide quick contact with medical care. Other doctors take their own patients' after-hours calls and see children at the hospital emergency room if they must be examined.

### Visiting the Pediatrician
Most pediatricians schedule your baby for an appointment about two weeks after birth. This may be a big day for you, a chance to show your baby off to a whole office filled with admiring people and an opportunity to ask all the questions that you have accumulated during this short time at home. Don't feel that anything is too "silly" to ask the doctor. If it has bothered you (or just left you feeling uncertain) it isn't silly and you will probably feel a lot better if you discuss it now. Some of the things you ask may not have one absolute answer. For instance, if you are wondering when to begin solid food or how long you should let your baby cry, you may find you encounter a variety of opinions. Some doctors will make specific suggestions based on their experience with many children. Others will present you with many options and tell you it is up to you which you choose—none will do any harm, and one just might work for you. First hint: This may be the first time you have gone out with your baby. Start getting ready at least thirty minutes before you would have if you were going by yourself. It can take an incredible amount of time to get the baby, the supplies, and yourself out the door! Second hint: Often the wait at the doctor's office is much longer than you anticipated. Bring diapers, a change of outfit for the baby, and a bottle if you are using them. As your child grows older, toys, books and drawing supplies can be helpful, not only in the waiting room, but also after you have been taken to the examining room.

# TAKING CARE OF OLDER CHILDREN

If you return home from your Cesarean to one or more older children, you face a special set of problems. First, your separation has been longer than if you had delivered vaginally. Even if your child was able to visit you briefly in the hospital, you were probably missed. You are still very tired and in some discomfort, which makes caring for older children more difficult. And last, no matter how well you prepared any older children for the birth of the baby, they probably will not have anticipated what is actually involved in sharing you with this tiny stranger.

### When You Have a Toddler

If you have a toddler, the logistics of caring for him after a Cesarean can be especially tricky. You probably have been told not to lift him during the first weeks after your delivery. If you had been using a changing table, you may find that a bed or a couch or the floor works much better now. If your toddler wants to be held, sit down on the floor next to him and take him on your lap. You may have to help your toddler learn to get in and out of bed and his high chair without as much assistance from you as he is used to. (Practical hints for working this out are in Chapter Thirteen, "Having Another Cesarean.") Usually you can accommodate to the restriction on lifting, but it may take a lot of ingenuity. It may also wear on your nerves.

> When I came home from the hospital with our second child, our oldest was about eighteen months old. The doctor said I was absolutely not to lift him. One evening shortly after I came home, my husband went to the store. Our eighteen month old woke in his crib and started to cry. I tried singing, patting, and changing his diaper. Nothing worked. All he wanted was a good snuggle. I remember trying to explain to him how to climb out of the crib after I put the side down. The poor kid was so confused! I was terrified to pick

him up, but I wanted to hold him right then more than anything in the whole world.

### Sharing Your Time

Often when you first return home, older children make demands of you that they never have before. They need to know that they are still loved and an important part of your family. They may choose unfortunate ways to let these feelings show.

> Every time I sat down to nurse the new baby, our two year old began to ask for something. It could be a drink of water, a toy, or a trip to the park. I felt trapped. I couldn't relax and just enjoy my time feeding the new baby and I couldn't respond to the needs of my two year old very well either. It all came home to me when our older child began answering everything with, "Just a minute. I busy." I must have said those same words to him hundreds of times during those first few weeks.

If you have someone to help during your first days at home, it is a good idea for you to be the one to take care of your older child. It is like walking a tightrope, trying to balance the needs of your older children, the new baby, and your own need for rest.

There are some things you can do to make life easier. Often you can look at a book with your older child while you are feeding the baby. He can turn the pages and you can read, or your older child can draw or do a puzzle right next to you. This way he has your attention, and your baby is snuggled and hears the sound of your voice. There are things that you and your older child can do together for the baby. Very young children usually enjoy helping to bathe the baby (although this tends to be a messy business and you should have lots of towels and superhuman patience if you try it!). They can also get diapers and toys for their new brother or sister. It is especially important that you find times alone for your older child or children. You can take walks, go to the park for a swing, or just sit and cuddle your older child. Sometimes you can even take a nap together while the baby sleeps—or at least get into bed together and look at a book. It may be very tempting to start the laundry or straighten the house while the baby is sleeping. If household chaos really gets on your nerves, perhaps your older child can "help" dust or fold the laundry.

As the weeks go by it is much easier if you can get both children on approximately the same schedule. Bathing two children at the same time is a lot less time-consuming than giving each her own bath. It is a lot simpler if your older child can eat while you are feeding the baby. The best relief of all is to have both children nap at the same time, but this is often something of "the impossible dream" for many mothers.

## Is This Sibling Rivalry?

> Brian seemed to have adjusted very well to the birth of his sister. He was warm and tender with her, but most of the time he was busy with his toys and his life. Then, a few weeks after she was born, he started hiding her pacifier at the bottom of his toybox. Other things of hers would "mysteriously" disappear. One night at bedtime, he asked me what was wrong with him. I said I didn't understand and he said that something must have been wrong with him if we thought we needed another baby.

Handling your older child's feelings about the new baby can seem like one problem too many when you are trying to cope with your own discomfort and fatigue following a Cesarean delivery. It can be difficult to remain calm in the face of a three year old who is threatening to throw a wooden truck on top of his sister. On the other hand, like all parents who have a second child, you want your firstborn to feel as loved and secure as he always has.

Although many parents prepare older children for a new baby, talk and reality are two different things. Almost all children experience some amount of difficulty once the baby comes to live at *their* house. It happens in most families and probably is not caused by something you are or are not doing. Your entire family is in a state of flux right now, and new ways of relating to one another will evolve with time.

There isn't one right way to help your older child adjust to a new baby. You can do as much as you can to assure him that he is still very important to you. You can share your happiness and exasperation about the new baby with him. Mostly, you can show that you love him. Each family finds ways that work (sometimes) for them.

I was really feeling smug. I told everyone that my children were the best of friends. Then one day, when Laurie was about two, I heard her screaming at our four year old son. She was just yelling her head off saying it was her truck and she wanted it back. Then she really let him have it! Smack! I then knew what sibling rivalry was all about.

## TAKING CARE OF YOUR MARRIAGE

The word "crisis" means a turning point or a crucial situation. The birth of your baby is a true crisis in your marriage. You are no longer two adults whose major responsibility is to one another. Where before there was one relationship, husband and wife, now there are three: husband and wife, wife and baby, husband and baby. Each relationship must develop by itself, while accommodating to the growth of the others in the family. Underlying all family interactions is the knowledge that this baby is totally dependent on both of you. An infant's needs cannot be ignored (postponed perhaps for a few minutes, but never absolutely ignored!). A lot of the energy and caring that used to flow between you will now be directed to your baby.

Often new parents wait for things to get back to normal after the baby is born. If "normal" means the way things were before you had the baby, this will just never happen. This doesn't mean that once you have made the transition into parenthood your life will be less than it was before. It will be different: richer, changed in ways that you might never have imagined.

Nick and I used to spend Saturday afternoons "exploring." We would go to bookstores or antiquing and have a late dinner at a new restaurant. After the baby was born, we just stopped going and we both missed those outings a lot. But we began to spend Sunday morning in bed—all three of us. One of us would get a light breakfast ready and bring food, the morning paper, and the baby back to bed. It felt so complete, so warm to be all together like that.

## A Woman, a Wife, a Mother

What does becoming a mother do to your feelings about yourself as a woman and a wife? At the simplest level it becomes one more way for you to define yourself. But you cannot separate the "mother" part of you from the "woman" or the "wife" parts. Gradually you adjust so that your life encompasses each role. You redefine yourself—a woman, a wife, and a mother—and are enriched by each role you have adopted.

When I first came home from the hospital with the baby, I felt so overwhelmed by being a MOTHER. I didn't seem to have any time for my husband or for myself either. I enjoyed taking care of the baby. I felt good feeding and bathing her. But I felt a little lost, too. I wondered what had happened to *me* in the midst of the diapers and the feedings. I worried about what was going on in my marriage. It took a long time, now that I look back on it, but I did find a sense of balance again. I found time to do things that I got a lot of satisfaction from, besides caring for Lisa. My husband and I "refound" one another, too. It was sort of like meeting all over again.

Sometimes a woman who has a Cesarean delivery has some strong feelings about her capabilities. Has she failed as a woman because she did not have a vaginal birth? If she "failed" at birth, will she also fail as a woman and as a wife? If you are feeling inadequate, you may shut your husband off from yourself and the baby. You may feel a variety of emotions when he offers you help. You may be trying to care for the baby without any help, in order to prove that you are a good mother. You may feel guilty because your husband is doing many of the things you usually do around the house and you just can't accept any more of his help. It may be very complex—a mixture of feelings about how a woman acts once she is a mother, a need to be in control of your life again, and some things you couldn't possibly verbalize.

At the same time you are coping with changing roles, you are going through a hormonal adjustment as your body returns to the nonpregnant state. You may find that you cry over very small things. Or you may get really angry about behavior that has never bothered you before.

> Jim always piled all his dishes in the sink after he used them. It meant that when I wanted to wash the dishes I had to take everything out before I could run the water. We had been doing this for two years but after the baby was born, it drove me crazy. I just erupted one night. He was absolutely astounded.

### A Man, a Husband, a Father

Fatherhood brings equally intense changes in the life of most men. They may be surprised at the tenderness they feel for this baby. Since many men did not grow up in a household where the father was directly involved in nurturing the children, their own feelings about the baby and their role in caring for him may cause them to redefine how they see themselves as a man.

A man may feel a sense of responsibility for his wife and child that is almost overwhelming for a time. The words "home" and "family" may take on added importance in his life. Some men may feel a certain sense of loss if their wives spend a great deal of the time they used to share together caring for the baby. They may feel shut out from the closeness between mother and child.

If your wife had a Cesarean delivery, you may feel some sense of failure or disappointment also. Were you enough support to her during labor? Did you miss something you can never make up for if you weren't present for the birth? Are you doing enough now to help at home?

There may be a conflict between the amount of time a man would like to spend at home and the hours he must be absent because of his job. It may be difficult, too, to come home to a somewhat frazzled household where something else always seems to be waiting for his attention.

I drove home from work one night wondering what we had done to ourselves. Why did we have this baby, anyway? Life was sure a lot simpler before. Then I walked in the door and Jane handed me this little bundle of a person. The baby and I sat and read the newspaper and I just felt so good. I guess life was simpler—but complications are great, too.

## Taking Time to Talk
This just isn't an easy time for either of you.

It took a long time before I could share the way I felt about the Cesarean and motherhood with Tom. For one thing, I felt guilty about how I felt. When I finally brought it up, he was really surprised. He had a hard time understanding that I was unhappy about the surgical birth and was lonely being home all day. I let it go for a while, but then we talked a couple more times. Even though I don't think he will ever really understand, he does know that I'm bothered and he listens when I need to talk.

There is a real value in sharing your feelings with one another. Even if you don't think the other person completely understands or even agrees with you, there are benefits for both of you if you feel free to talk about what is bothering you—or what is bringing you particular joy, for that matter. Sometimes it is easier to spend your time taking care of your baby rather than discussing what is happening in your lives. You both have needs and you both have responsibilities toward each other and toward your baby. The more open you can be with one another about this complex business of parenthood, the easier adjustment period you will have.

## Sharing the Responsibility
Just as you chose to have this baby together, you can now decide how you will take care of your child together. The ways of parenting together are really endless and all have benefits. The important point is that you discuss how you are going to go about it, rather than fall into patterns without examining why you are doing what you are doing. Couples sometimes make assumptions about how each partner views parenthood. They may not stop long enough to feel out how each of them is responding to the re-

sponsibilities of having a baby. Each of us has ideas about what being a mother or a father entails, based primarily on our experience with our own parents. When we become parents ourselves, we may find that some of these preconceived notions don't fit with our present life or with our partner's expectations.

Once you have worked out your own system of "coparenting" you will need to respect one another's actions and decisions about your baby. There will probably be times when you disagree about some aspect of child care. If your lines of communication are open, you can work toward a compromise that will be comfortable to both of you. There will be times when you will have to relinquish your feelings about "the proper way" to do a particular task and respect your partner's right to do things his or her way.

> I had a very set way of giving the baby her bath. My mother had always told me that you wash a baby's face first and then work your way down the body. When Bill bathed the baby, he just washed her any old way. I always wanted to run right up, grab the washcloth, and tell him I would do it the RIGHT WAY. It took me a long time, but I finally learned that on his days to bathe Beth he did it his way. When we chose to share taking care of her, I gave up my right to be the only resident expert on child care.

### Making Some Adjustments

Even if you are sharing responsibility for your baby, you will still need time for just yourselves. Sometimes you have to make rather major adjustments in your lifestyle so you can still have this time once your baby is born. You may find that rearranging some of your routines will accomplish some of this—for instance, sharing laundry or dish duty rather than having one of you do each job. If your baby is lively and wants to be fed, held, and played with at six o'clock, when you used to have dinner, perhaps you can share a light snack then and have dinner later, when the baby is sleeping again. Be realistic, however. If the thought of fixing dinner at seven-thirty and doing dishes at nine makes both of you cringe, this plan will not work for you. Nor will it work if you have a baby who stays awake from 4:00 P.M. to midnight.

It is important that you get out together without the baby sometimes, too. After a Cesarean, you may not feel like getting dressed up and leaving your home for a while, but the time will come. Finding a reliable baby sitter can be one of life's major problems. Perhaps you have a neighbor or relative who will help you at the beginning. Some communities have baby sitting co-operatives where parents take turns caring for each other's children and earn baby sitting time rather than money. You can also ask friends to recommend sitters they have used. Often colleges or senior high schools have lists of people who are interested in part-time baby sitting. Some cities have professional baby sitting agencies. These services are frequently more expensive than someone you hire directly. Such agencies usually provide older, experienced people, however, and this may be helpful if you are feeling unsure about leaving your child.

While your baby is small you can still get out by taking him with you to many places. A light, portable crib is helpful at these times. Picnics, dinner at a friend's home, even shopping expeditions provide a chance for all of you to get out of the house for a while. This only works until your baby begins spending more time awake than asleep or until he becomes vitally interested in what is going on around him!

## Sex After a Cesarean

After a time one or both of you will wish to resume sexual relations. Although most doctors suggest that you do not have intercourse until after your six-week checkup, some couples find it difficult to wait this length of time. Other couples wait the full six weeks or much longer. A lot will depend on how the woman is feeling both physically and emotionally.

If you are tired and uncomfortable following your Cesarean, worries about sexual matters may be the farthest thing from your mind. If you do think about it, you may be afraid that intercourse will hurt. Or it may be hard to believe that your mate really desires your intimacy when you are having trouble thinking of yourself as a beautiful woman. A scar on the abdomen, shaved pubic hair, and a collection of stretch marks may not do much for your self-concept. You may not be thinking of yourself as unattractive but rather as changed. There is a loss of innocence that can accompany the birth of a baby that many women find difficult to overcome. You may feel that you have been poked, prodded, and entered by so many people in the past few weeks that you need time to regain control of your own body before you can share it with your husband again.

Although the feelings may not be as intense, a man may have reservations about intercourse, also. He may worry that he will hurt his mate. He may have some feelings about her role as mother, and this will change his perception of this woman as his sex partner for a time.

In addition to these problems, you are both probably tired during these first few months. You are getting up to feed your baby during the night. Then there is always the fear that just at a crucial moment in your love-making, the baby will wake up. Neither the thought of getting up to take care of the baby nor the prospect of trying to continue while the baby cries is very appealing.

Your need to be close physically will return. Since the hormonal changes that occur in the postpartum period often affect a woman's level of sexual desire, you may find that you just are not as responsive to your mate as you were before the baby was born. Of course, these desires will return, but many women are surprised that it can take six months or more before they really feel interested in responding to their mate. There are some things that you can do to make this time easier and indeed pleasurable for both of you. Many couples find that other kinds of intimacy —fondling and genital stimulation, for example—avoid the psychological and physical pressures that might be implied in intercourse. If you do wish to have intercourse, it is often more comfortable for the woman to be on top or next to the man rather than using the man-on-top or missionary position. There usually is a reduction in vaginal lubrication after the birth of a baby, which can make intercourse uncomfortable if you are unprepared. You can avoid this problem by using a lubricating gel (such as KY) specifically designed for this purpose.

If you do have intercourse, make sure you use some method of birth control. You can become pregnant again right after you have a baby, even if you are breast-feeding. Until you see your doctor and decide on a permanent method of birth control, use at least a condom and perhaps a spermicidal foam each time you have intercourse.

### Giving Yourself Time

Your sexual relationship is much more complex than the time you spend in bed together. The physical enjoyment that can be had from sexual intimacy is important, of course. But this kind of intimacy is also a way of saying to each other, "I really value you." We cannot give a blueprint for how you will do this in your marriage. We can suggest that you avoid putting pressure on yourself or your partner. Try to accept how you are feeling right now without being concerned about two weeks or two months from now. Communicate as much as you are comfortable doing. Most of all, give yourselves time. You will find ways of relating to one another, perhaps through intercourse, or perhaps by the briefest of hugs, that will communicate the love you are feeling for each other.

# TEN

# Your Emotional Responses to Cesarean Birth

You and your baby have come through a lot together. For this reason, a baby born by surgical delivery can be a special delight. Although all couples experience joy in having their baby, parental response to the actual Cesarean birth process varies greatly.

Some couples who have Cesareans find the birth of their baby totally rewarding. Probably the most satisfied couples are the ones who know of their Cesarean long enough in advance to become prepared. Even as little as five years ago, there were almost no books to read or classes to take to get ready for a Cesarean birth. Now many more doctors tell their patients in advance to be prepared for either mode of delivery, and the opportunities to read and learn about Cesarean birth are rapidly increasing. Preparation increases the confidence of parents and encourages acceptance of even the most difficult aspects of birth.

When he first said it would have to be a Cesarean, I went home and cried. I was scared to get cut up and scared that something would go wrong. But I got the name of someone in the Cesarean group and we went to a meeting. It turned out that they had some slides of a Cesarean. When I saw them, then I knew I could do it.

Most couples have mixed feelings about their Cesarean birth. There is the relief and joy of having your baby, no matter how she got here. Yet other feelings come and go, feelings that conflict with that relief and joy. And, of course, there are the rapid emotional shifts of any pregnancy and postpartum period. You may be elated about your baby in the morning, worried about your scar in the afternoon, and just plain exhausted by dinnertime.

Mixed feelings are perfectly normal and natural. The positive feelings that parents have about childbirth don't come as surprises to anyone. But the negative feelings aren't so easy to accept. Does everyone have negative feelings about their childbirth experience? Yes, almost everyone has some. And there is reason to believe that Cesarean couples who have little or no time to prepare have more negative feelings about the birth experience than do couples who are prepared.

For some couples, the negative responses to a Cesarean are very strong. They have planned, practiced, and invested themselves emotionally in a shared vaginal birth. The sense of loss they feel is very great, and their ways of expressing their feelings are similar to the ways in which people express grief over other kinds of losses.

I felt assaulted—raped, perhaps, by what had happened to my body with absolutely no control on my part. I had gone through Lamaze classes twice, I had had a vaginal delivery the first time, and I knew what I was going to do this time too. But nothing went the way it was supposed to.

If you have negative feelings about your Cesarean, whether they are minor or very great indeed, you are not abnormal and you are certainly not alone. Below are some of the most common negative responses to Cesarean birth, and suggestions about how to cope with them.

## SCARED

Naturally! Most people have some fear of the surgery itself, and often there are fears about the anesthetic as well. (In addition, the very fact that surgery is being performed may mean that there is reason to be afraid for the baby's health, the mother's, or both.) And, of course, it is frightening to be in a strange situation, probably not at all like what you prepared for. In some hospitals, Cesarean mothers must be moved to a new floor where the surgical suite is located for the actual birth. If you have relied on the support of certain maternity staff during labor, this move into the hands of strangers can increase your fear. And since most hospitals still don't allow husbands to be present for Cesarean deliveries, many husbands report feeling scared on their wife's behalf, while wives worry about how the banished husband is doing.

The scared feeling often goes away as soon as the surgery is over. But if you have never had surgery before, there may be some parts of your recovery that seem scary too, such as the first walk after the birth. These events are routine to the nurses who are supporting you, so feel free to let them in on how you are feeling.

Some parents continue to worry about whether their baby is really healthy. After all, if your doctor couldn't predict your Cesarean, can he really predict the baby's well-being? This is a normal response to being thrown into an unexpected situation.

If you are having continuing fears about what happened to you and whether the baby is healthy, or if you have tremendous fear of another Cesarean even though you want another child, then you need to do some work to inform and educate yourself. Reading and talking to others can help you put such fears in better perspective.

## HELPLESS

This feeling is most common among couples who have had child-birth preparation classes. During labor, the woman is very busy and active. You have trained yourself to concentrate and remain in control as much as you can. Your husband is equally busy, timing contractions, counting for you, giving back rubs and leg rubs, and communicating with the hospital staff. But with a Cesarean delivery, particularly one that is not planned, you find yourself having things done to you, rather than your doing them.

> After the birth of our first child, I felt incomplete. We worked so hard together, and it seemed to go so well at first. Then everything was stopped and the baby was taken from me. I didn't have the good feeling of resolution, of feeling my baby leave my body.

Your husband, meanwhile, is commonly left in the old traditional role of pacing around the waiting room. He is unable to help you at a time when each of you may feel you need each other the most.

Afterward, particularly if you have never had surgery before, there may be a period of feeling helpless as a parent. How can you mother this frail new baby when you cannot even get to the bathroom on your own? The normal doubts you have about yourself as a mother may become temporarily quite exaggerated. Perhaps everything goes along well enough while you are hospitalized. But are they really going to send you home and expect you to care for that baby? And the new father, who may have little experience caring for a baby, is now expected to support a wife who is trying to recover from surgery, as well as to take care of the baby while she rests.

Although you gain new strength with each day, you are right to think of yourself as having some real physical and emotional limitations, probably greater than any you have felt before. Most of us don't like that helpless feeling, but this is no time to pull out the Superwoman routine either. You need and deserve support, and while you are still in the hospital is the time to start planning for who will help you at home, if you have not already made these arrangements. It is realistic to expect that you will be able to take on a major share of the baby's care when you go home from the hospital, provided you do *nothing* else. Give in to that helpless feeling and let others take over for you.

Husbands, too, deserve to be taken care of while learning to care for a newly dependent wife and baby. Beg, borrow, steal, or hire help now!

## RESENTFUL, ANGRY

When something goes wrong, or doesn't go the way you planned, it is natural to search for someone to hold responsible for what happened. You may feel that your doctor caused you a lot of unnecessary problems by not preparing you for your Cesarean far in advance. You may be angry at your childbirth instructor for what, in retrospect, seems like very limited coverage of Cesarean birth in the classes you attended. Some women become resigned to the birth itself, but then get angry at the nursing staff for the pain that must be endured during the recovery period. You may feel resentful toward your baby for putting you through the trauma of surgical birth.

To some extent, your ability to talk about these feelings will depend on how "legitimate" they seem to you.

> The whole thing made me just furious. I was mad at the doctor, my husband, and most of all myself. I couldn't sort it out. When one of the nurses didn't answer the call bell for ten minutes, I almost enjoyed the excuse to let off some steam. I really lit into her for leaving me lying there.

If you can identify what is making you angry, then you are more likely to express yourself. If you aren't sure what angers you, then you may think that you have to keep your feelings to yourself.

This can create serious problems, however, as resentments build up inside you with no outlet. It is probably better to express your feelings, regardless of whether you think they are justified. If you can talk about feeling angry without making the other person feel attacked, so much the better. Sometimes it helps to talk out your feelings with some neutral but understanding person before you talk directly to the person at whom you are angry.

It may also help you to think about what support you need or actions you can take to help you feel more comfortable and cared for. Perhaps some additional information about why things happened the way they did would help. One woman just started writing down everything about her birth experience that bothered her. She waited until she had gone home and settled into a routine, and then composed a very well-thought-out letter to her doctor and the hospital maternity staff that actually resulted in some policy changes. Although it didn't change what happened to her, her anger was tempered by a real sense of achievement.

Once you leave the hospital, particularly during the extended period of your physical recovery, each parent may experience anger at or resentment of the demands made by the other, and by the baby. These feelings are not uncommon, regardless of how the baby is born. But if you have a Cesarean birth, you have less energy to bring to this first part of parenthood. The more tired you are, the more likely you are to resent the demands of your new situation and the apparent failure of your partner fully to understand or support you.

Your needs are no less important than your baby's. The difference is that you can postpone meeting your own needs in order to care for your baby. But be sure to plan time for yourselves, when each of you can be taken care of too. This is especially important when your formal helper has left and you are all by yourselves as a family. If you do not feel comfortable leaving the baby for a whole evening, you may enjoy just an hour with your feet up while a neighborhood teen-ager takes the baby for a walk. Each of you needs time to get away alone and time to be together without interruption.

## DISAPPOINTED, SAD

Couples who have taken childbirth preparation classes are almost invariably disappointed that things did not turn out the way they hoped. Feeling this way does not mean that you love your baby any less. It simply means that you hoped, planned, and practiced for a particular way of bringing this baby into the world, and now you have lost that hoped-for experience. Like life's other turning points, you wanted everything to be just right. If you had some warning, or planned for a variety of types of birth from the start, then you may not feel such an acute sense of loss. But if you had your heart set on an "awake and aware" childbirth, then your actual birth experience was probably a far cry from your dreams, and you may be very sorrowful about what you have lost. Or if you had no strong preconceived notions about the details of the delivery, but counted on being together, your sense of being cheated out of sharing one of life's beautiful moments may remain for some time.

> For a while, I thought I was crazy to feel like this. My husband thought I was making a mountain out of a molehill. I didn't even try to explain it to my doctor. Now that I have talked to other Cesarean mothers, I can finally say it clearly: I love my baby, but I hate the way she got here.

Since there is no going back, the only solution for strong feelings of disappointment is to find things to enjoy in the present while you also look forward. It helps to talk about your feelings to each other, and to other Cesarean couples who will understand your disappointment. It may help to get involved in a Cesarean support group or to work on getting Cesarean childbirth preparation classes started in your area. You can ease some of the disappointment by starting now to do the work that will make your next Cesarean—or someone else's—more satisfying.

I still feel lingering moments of sadness, focused mostly on the fact that I will never know what it is like to push the baby out myself. The feelings come back whenever another friend has a baby. But most of the time, I hardly think about it anymore.

## ALONE, WITHDRAWN

There is the literal aloneness if you were separated from your husband during your baby's birth. When you thought the birth would be vaginal, you wanted to be together to share the joy of that moment. If the birth must be a Cesarean, many couples want to be together even more. If your Cesarean is a surprise, you won't have time to change the policy if your hospital does not allow fathers to attend surgical births. For couples who have time to plan and prepare, finding ways to share the birth may become an essential aspect of the planning process (see Chapter Fourteen, "Father-Attended Cesarean Birth").

Later there is the feeling of being alone, which you may have when you compare notes with friends or relatives whose children were born vaginally. All of us deal with our experiences to some degree by talking to others and identifying what we have in common. As Cesarean parents, you may be reluctant to share your birth experience with others, particularly if they seem put off by the talk about surgery, or if they are just out of touch with what you are saying and feeling. Yet you need to tell about what happened to you, as all new parents do.

Both of Marie's girls weighed more than ten pounds when they were born. I guess her delivery was rough both times, but it didn't seem as bad to me that way as having a Cesarean. She is a good friend and I thought she would understand my feelings. But when I told her that I was disappointed about having a Cesarean, she just shrugged and made some crack like, "Honey, you didn't miss a thing!" She meant it to be funny, I guess.

Some Cesarean parents keep their birth experiences to themselves because they are reluctant to admit that there were some very unpleasant parts of the birth. If you think you are supposed to feel wholeheartedly delighted by something, you may choose to keep your misgivings to yourself.

If you have had a Cesarean already, be sure to take time to sit down and share all of your memories of the experience with each other. In addition, couples who have had Cesareans particularly enjoy sharing their birth experience with other Cesarean couples. Look around—you're not alone!

## INADEQUATE, A FAILURE

> I have always been able to do things if I really put my mind to it. And anyone can have a baby, right? Thousands of women do it every day. Nature just proceeds, with maybe a small assist from the woman and her doctor. Except all of a sudden it was my turn, and I couldn't do it. Having a baby, the simplest, most natural thing in the world, and I couldn't do it.

The sense of inadequacy or failure is more common among women. To some degree, each of us feels that our womanliness is connected to our bodies, and particularly to our ability to have children. If you don't deliver your children the "normal" way, then you may feel that you are less of a woman. Your husband, too, may feel that you "should" be able to have the baby vaginally—as though it were in your power to change whatever factors caused your surgical birth!

Some fathers feel inadequate when they are asked to leave before the birth. If you are a husband who placed a strong value on supporting your wife through labor and delivery, then you may feel that you have failed her in some way by not being there for the delivery. Yet this was not something you could change, any more than your wife could change the fact that the baby could not be born vaginally.

Our worth as people and as parents has no relationship to the way our children came into the world. To be sure, if you looked forward to the baby's arrival for most of the past nine months, then it is entirely normal to have a sense of failure when some major portion of the experience does not go as planned. Some women find that breast-feeding their baby is enough to overcome their initial sense of failure. For other parents, feelings of success and competence return when the recovery from surgery is well along and they are engrossed in parenthood.

## DEPRESSED

It's hard to say exactly how you feel when you're depressed. It's the blues, feeling low and tired, uneasy or dissatisfied. Depression is very common after having a baby. The causes are both hormonal and psychological. But if you have a Cesarean birth, your normal depression may be magnified by the physical shock to your body, and by your feelings about your birth experience.

In addition to waiting for yourself to start feeling better, which you will, you can take some steps to help yourself. Get as much rest as possible. It may be hard to force yourself to sit down or lie down, especially after a few weeks, when what you really want to do is get going on life again. But your body is still physically depleted and needs your tender, loving care. If your helpers have all left, your friends can make casseroles or your neighbor can watch the baby for a little while. Find ways to get out of the house often, but don't overdo it. An overambitious grocery shopping trip may leave you feeling even worse than before. But a short walk around the block will help to remind you that the world is still out there waiting for you.

For some reason, it often is hard to talk about your feelings when you are depressed. Yet this can be the best therapy of all. There is probably at least one person who is close to you—your husband, another relative, or a friend—who would feel honored that you trust him or her enough to share your most personal thoughts and feelings. And as you talk, you will find yourself feeling relieved and exploring ways to resolve your depression.

## GUILTY

You have just had a surprise Cesarean birth. You are searching for some explanation, some justification. Almost all of us have some notion that the world is a just place and people get what they deserve sooner or later. So what did you do to deserve this?

Absolutely nothing! Your Cesarean was not caused by your gaining ten pounds more than the doctor said to, or working right up to your due date, or eating too much pizza just before you went into labor. Nor was it caused by your losing control after nine hours of labor. You would have had a Cesarean even if you had not missed one of your childbirth preparation classes. In other words, you do not "deserve" this Cesarean, in the sense of being paid back for some mistake you made.

Husbands, too, express feelings of guilt.

> During those first twenty-four hours, it looked to me like she was suffering a lot. I had never seen anyone who just had an operation before, so I didn't know she would feel much better in a short while. I just knew she was in pain, and I had a part in causing the pregnancy and the pain. I had the crazy wish that I could take some of the pain myself, equal up the burden somehow.

Probably the best therapy for guilt is to find out as much as you can about what caused your Cesarean. Don't hesitate to ask your doctor to explain more than once. There may be much that your doctor does not know either, but the facts that can be known will help you accept your Cesarean without guilt.

## JEALOUS

> At first, I thought my roommate was the luckiest person in the world. She got her baby right away, and she walked around without bending over, and she seemed to have so much energy. Plus I kept

having to listen while she told all her friends how the baby was born. Seven hours of labor, almost no medication. It just didn't seem fair.

It is certainly normal to envy someone who apparently has something that you wished for and worked for. These feelings are often stronger when your birth experience is recent and you are feeling at your weakest. As time goes by and your baby thrives in much the same way as your roommate's, then the issue of how the baby arrived becomes much less important. Sometimes friends who have delivered vaginally will understand your jealousy; or, focusing on the ways in which childbirth and parenthood were not perfect for them either, they may take the position that you have nothing to complain about. It helps to share your feelings with other Cesarean parents.

## WHEN YOU NEED HELP

Most parents find that talking together, taking steps to help themselves feel better, and the passage of time all combine to help them achieve a new perspective on their birth experience. A Cesarean that came as a bitter disappointment does not ever seem wonderful, but it does become less important as the adventure of parenthood becomes a reality. For a few parents, however, the negative feelings do not subside. Then it is time to consult your physician, clergyman, or a mental health professional.

How do you decide whether you need help? There is no exact way to measure yourself or make this decision. It is entirely normal for the postpartum period to be a time of upheaval, so you might expect at least several months of emotional uproar in your lives. After allowing for that, there are several guidelines that may be helpful in assessing your situation. If you can see obvious ways in which your feelings about the birth are interfering either with your ability to be a good parent or your relationship with your partner, then an outside viewpoint may be in order. If there is a large gap between the way things are actually going in the family and your beliefs about how things realistically ought to be, then you may need some professional help in resolving the differences. Sometimes the best way to decide if you need professional help is simply to go to one or more professionals and ask for their opinion.

## ACCEPTANCE

You have not just had a baby. You have had a baby *and* major abdominal surgery. You will regain your strength and spirits more slowly than women who have delivered vaginally. You may find that you still feel like you are undergoing the postpartum adjustment period far beyond the traditional six to eight weeks. A great deal of your ability to enjoy your new baby during this time will depend on your having realistic expectations for yourself.

Acceptance comes with time and is helped by your willingness to examine and express your feelings about this birth and this baby. There are no "wrong" feelings, although there are sometimes uncomfortable feelings and unsympathetic listeners. Some people, like your doctor and your husband, need to hear what you are feeling regardless of whether they are sympathetic from the start. Please be patient but persistent in talking to them, and in listening.

Sometimes parents become aware that they have accepted their first Cesarean when they have gone through a second birth that is more positive. It is as though the chance to "do it right" brings the ability to put aside feelings about the first Cesarean.

Acceptance sometimes disappears after it has arrived. You may feel as though you have completely resolved all your feelings about the birth, only to have them reappear when an unmedicated vaginal birth is shown on TV, or your friend shows you the pictures of her easy, prepared birth in the local hospital's birthing room. Being reminded of what you missed can bring some of the old feelings back, but they will drift away again.

Often Cesarean parents are told, "Having a healthy baby is all that matters." This trite phrase has a hollow ring to the woman whose disappointment about having surgery is very fresh, or to the father who feels cheated because he could not greet his child at birth. But for some parents, the stage of acceptance begins when they can say, "Having a healthy baby really is all that matters." For others, the regrets that accompany the birth continue to coexist with the enjoyment that the baby brings.

> When Dana had his first birthday, I naturally got to remembering the day he was born. As I thought about it, I realized that I hadn't been wishing "If only it could have been different" for a long time. I guess I stopped fighting the reality and accepted it. I had a Cesarean. It isn't what I wanted, but it is what happened. So be it.

# ELEVEN

# Parent-Infant Bonding

You probably heard the word "bonding" mentioned in your childbirth preparation classes or read it in the popular literature for parents. You may even have planned your birth experience to include some special time together as a family right after the baby's birth, so that you could begin the bonding process immediately. If you had an unexpected Cesarean instead, you more than likely had a quick glimpse of the baby at birth, or a first visit after your anesthesia wore off and you were feeling very uncomfortable. Neither meeting was the way you imagined that your family would begin.

Even if you are able to plan your Cesarean birth, it is unlikely that your introduction to your baby will be picture-perfect. Since in this case you have time to plan, you should investigate what the usual practices are in your area. If you can have a regional anesthetic, and if both parents can be together for the birth or in the recovery room immediately afterward, then many of your hopes for early contact can be fulfilled. Many Cesarean parents want to touch and hold the baby as soon as possible, and to avoid separation unless there is a medical reason. Of course, this requires that the father or other support person be allowed to take care of the baby in the mother's room until she is able to do so herself. If these options are not currently available in your area, your doctor and hospital may be willing to consider them for your baby's upcoming birth.

The popularity of the idea of bonding stems mostly from the work of Drs. Marshall H. Klaus and John H. Kennell, who published their book *Maternal-Infant Bonding* in 1976. Klaus and Kennell were interested in the fact that some mothers of premature babies had trouble loving and caring for their babies, even when the baby was finally declared healthy and ready to come home. If something could go wrong, Klaus and Kennell theorized, then there might be some normal process of attachment between parents and infants that usually went right. But what was it? How do parents fall in love with their babies?

> My mother always told me how she knew I was the right baby even though they didn't let her see me until two days after I was born, because I had curly hair and Grandma Long's eyes. I loved to hear that story about my arrival. It wasn't until I was a parent myself that I realized that she couldn't really have known if my eyes would be like Grandma Long's. I guess she thought it was true at the time. I think it was her way of learning to love me and make me hers.

In their most familiar studies, Klaus and Kennell focused on the effects of separating mothers and babies at birth. Twenty-eight mothers were randomly assigned to one of two groups. Fourteen of the mothers had the amount of contact with their newborn that was typical when the study was done (a glimpse of the baby at birth, a brief contact six or eight hours later, then feedings every four hours). The other fourteen mothers were given "early and extended contact" (having the nude baby in bed with them for one hour during the first two hours after birth, and having the baby with them for five extra hours on each of the remaining days in the hospital). The study demonstrated that the two groups of mothers behaved quite differently toward their babies during observations a month after the baby's birth, and also during observations when the babies were one and then two years old. For instance, the mothers who had had more contact with their babies fondled them more and were more likely to stand close and help the doctor while the baby was given a physical examination. Additional studies have been done of some of the children themselves, and these show that the "extended contact" children have higher IQs and scored higher on two language tests at age five than the children whose mothers had only the traditional amount of contact.

Many studies of a similar nature have now been completed, with the "early and extended contact" beginning at some time during the first three days after birth, though not always in the first hours after birth. On the basis of these studies, early contact is said to contribute to more successful breast-feeding, fewer infections, better weight gain, and even reductions in the number of children who are battered.

Specific "attachment behaviors" have been identified, and most mothers greeting their babies for the first time exhibit similar behaviors, in the same sequence. Some early studies seem to show that fathers act much like mothers when they first see their newborns, and also report very similar feelings to mothers'.

## THE PROBLEM OF SOCIOECONOMIC FACTORS

A major area of difficulty with this research that is often overlooked is that most of the mothers who were studied were coping with serious economic and social problems of their own. For instance, the mothers in Klaus and Kennell's study had an average age of slightly more than eighteen years when their babies were born. Two thirds of the mothers were not married. Based on objective criteria, the mothers lived in substandard housing and held unskilled jobs. Most had not reached the eleventh grade in school. Twenty-six of the twenty-eight mothers were black, meaning they were struggling against the effects of racism as well. Clearly, these mothers had critical needs of their own, and limited resources left over to devote to the care of their newborn.

What is really significant, therefore, is that none of the mothers who had extended contact appeared to have any difficulty becoming attached to their babies. The fact that early and extended contact had a positive impact is important because it shows that there are relatively simple ways to provide significant support to mothers who are otherwise statistically likely to have difficulty mothering. However, the research does not demonstrate what the effects of early and extended contact are for mothers of a different socioeconomic status, whose own needs presumably were being met to a greater degree before the birth of the baby. We may guess that early and extended contact would benefit almost all parents and babies. The new professional support for family-centered maternity care is a formal recognition of this benefit. But there is no evidence that separation of middle class mothers and babies does any lasting harm.

There are some studies of the effects of separation on middle class mothers and babies. Unfortunately, the separations occurred because the babies were sick and needed varying degrees of special care. This makes it impossible to determine whether the differences that were uncovered were due to the separation or to the baby's condition and the mother's response to it. One such study shows initial differences in both mothers and babies when there had been a separation lasting between two and fourteen days, as compared to mothers and babies who were not separated. Interestingly enough, most of the differences between the two groups had disappeared by the time the babies were three or four months old.

## NO MORE "CRITICAL PERIOD"

In their book, Klaus and Kennell devoted a great deal of attention to their theory that there was a critical period immediately after birth during which parents had to have contact with their infant in order for the baby to develop to her fullest potential. The existence of a life-threatening critical period in other mammals has been studied for many years. Some animals who are separated from their young for even short periods of time will completely reject the babies when they are reunited. Although no similar period for human beings is known, Klaus and Kennell have directed some of their efforts toward identifying a "critical period" in humans where the mother's feelings of attachment to her baby were either brought to their fullest through early contact, or interfered with in some way by separation in the first few days of the baby's life. There is a large body of evidence against the notion of any sort of critical period for human beings. Despite this, some parents and professionals too still believe that there is only one right way and only one right time to begin getting to know the baby.

What Klaus and Kennell suggest is that attachment is a complicated series of processes that all blend together over an extended period of time. They theorize that there are as many as fifty or sixty "switches" that get parents "turned on" to their baby, and they do not believe that every switch must be thrown at precisely a crucial moment in order for parents to feel the greatest possible attachment to their baby. The process of becoming attached often begins even before the mother feels the baby moving inside her, and continues long after the baby is born. In fact, defining and redefining that attachment is probably a lifelong process.

> I am petite—at least when I'm not pregnant!—and I pictured a little girl with my small size and her father's dark hair. Well, I was right about the hair. When I saw the baby the first few times it was hard to relate to him, and when I held him the first time—he was this nine-pound stranger. Now he crawls all over the apartment and I feel like I've known him forever.

There is some evidence to suggest that a newborn whose mother has not been medicated during labor and delivery remains quite alert and aware of her surroundings for a large part of the first hours after birth. The parents who see their baby this way are very likely to be completely captivated by the baby. They respond in ways that encourage the baby to respond even more to them, through looking at them and making cooing sounds, as well as in more subtle ways. This time is not a critical period in the true sense, although it may be appropriate to see it as a potentially sensitive period for some parents and babies. The family with a Cesarean birth is in a very different situation from the family with a vaginal birth when the mother has had no medication. The Cesarean baby may be a little sleepy right after birth, and her periods of being very responsive to her surroundings may be postponed until well after the first hour of life. The mother is coping with the effects of anesthesia and the surgery itself, while the father must deal with his heightened concerns for his wife's well-being as well as the baby's.

Even when the Cesarean is a planned, family centered event, the circumstances of the birth are different in many respects from those of an unmedicated vaginal delivery. There is no valid research on the significance of these differences. But common sense and experience tell us that Cesarean parents form a bond with their babies that is no different from the bond between parents and vaginally delivered babies.

Another argument against the "critical period" notion is the interesting study by Dr. Aidan MacFarlane, which looked at the question of when mothers reported first feeling love for their baby. Less than half of the mothers felt their first feelings of love during pregnancy. About one quarter of the mothers placed their first feelings of love for the baby at the time of birth, and many of the remainder identified the baby's first week of life as the time when they first felt love. Somewhat surprisingly, fully 12 per cent of the mothers said that they first felt love for their baby some time after the first week of life. One implication of MacFarlane's study is that the normal timetable for attachment to begin is quite varied. MacFarlane also discovered that about two-thirds of the mothers could identify specific points at which their love for the baby increased. This suggests something that probably all mothers know, which is that feelings of attachment build gradually, rather than simply arriving one day in a bundle brought by the stork.

## THE QUESTION OF VALUES

It is difficult to do research that does not reflect the values of the researchers. It is also difficult to present the results of research to the public without having people misinterpret the meaning of data. In their book, Klaus and Kennell say,

> These methods were designed to measure attachment and not to evaluate good or bad mothering.

Yet parents everywhere have thought that Klaus and Kennell proved that early contact is essential if you want to be a good parent.

It is also difficult to design ways merely to measure the existence of something called "attachment behaviors." Even if their existence can be measured, the question of whether "more attachment" means "better parenting" is still very much open to discussion. For instance, Klaus and Kennell interviewed the mothers in their study when the babies were about one month old. Among other questions, they asked if the mother had gone out since the baby was born, and if so, how she felt when she was away from the baby. A score of 3 points, or the greatest amount of attachment, was given if the mother did not go out without the baby, or if she did go out but thought about the baby constantly. A score of 0, the least amount of attachment, was given if the mother answered that she had been out and that she felt good and did not think about the baby while she was gone.

The trouble is that some women who are superb mothers feel very hemmed in by their newborn at times. As a result, they may be elated when a chance to run to the drugstore *alone* turns up. And some women who are not such superb mothers find it very hard to leave their babies—perhaps because they have so many doubts about themselves as mothers that they need their babies constantly nearby to reassure them.

My neighbor would leave her two kids with me once in a while and just go shopping. I was glad to help out. I never thought much about what it meant to her. Then I had Angie and I realized what it felt like to have that responsibility twenty-four hours a day. I decided to go volunteer somewhere once a week while my neighbor watched Angie, and it was wonderful.

## HOW MUCH DOES BONDING MATTER?

Klaus and Kennell have done an important service for parents by calling attention to the ways in which traditional medical practices may interfere with the natural process of becoming a family. Unfortunately, their results sometimes have been reported uncritically, or have been emphasized to the exclusion of all the other factors that make up the process of pregnancy, birth, and development of the child. In fact, Dr. Klaus is disturbed that the reporting of the research on bonding is encouraging parents to think that they must have immediate contact with their babies at birth, before the "glue" dries and all is lost.

We chose the hospital across town because it has a birthing room. My sister's second baby was born there and it just sounded so wonderful. They had pictures of her nursing the baby right after he was born. Naturally, I pictured that Christopher's birth would be that way too. When I had to have a Cesarean, it changed everything. I kept worrying about what it would mean and whether we had lost something precious. But when Christopher started nursing, I knew we would be OK. It was just a wonderful feeling and it felt so natural and right that I stopped worrying.

The benefits of early and extended contact may become clearer with this analogy: Women who are anemic benefit from iron supplements. Women who are not anemic may choose to take iron as a preventive measure. But if iron becomes unavailable, they will do fine without it. Early contact can be beneficial, but it is not essential.

We need to know more about what helps parents everywhere to

nurture children. Of special interest to the Cesarean parent will be studies of how we, who experience early separation and other stresses, come to experience the same joys and make the same mistakes that all parents do.

## AM I A GOOD PARENT?

How did you become the kind of parent you are? How did your child become the kind of person he is becoming? We are not even close to being able to answer these questions. We do know that a rich array of present circumstances and past events plays some part. Among the factors that we know have some influence are: the kind of parents your parents were; your baby's health at birth; your socioeconomic status; the kinds of stresses occurring in your family during your pregnancy and right after the baby's birth; the sex of the baby and whether she is the firstborn or not; and the kinds of social support you have when you come home with the baby.

Sometimes parents are so eager to do a good job of parenting that they lose sight of themselves. There are so many "experts" these days, and it can be either discouraging or reassuring to learn how limited our scientific knowledge is, and how much the experts disagree. For instance, although the concern about the first hours of life has become popular only recently, there has been a strong emphasis on the first year of life for many decades. Leading theorists have seemed to say that the personality of the child is written in stone in those first twelve months. Now, however, the emphasis is shifting toward the potential for continuing growth and development of the person throughout his or her life. Suddenly each individual is seen as someone who can grow and change, despite the joys or hardships of his or her first year.

Becoming attached and continuing to feel attached to your children is hard work. Often there are obstacles to overcome. If you wanted your first hours with your baby to be spent a particular way and they were not, then you are entitled to feel disappointed at the very least. You have lost something that you expected to treasure all your lives. But there is no evidence that your relationship with your baby has suffered any permanent damage.

Probably the real meaning of all the research on bonding is this: Parents, like babies, deserve as much support and approval as possible. By giving parents early and extended contact, hospitals are saying to parents, "We believe in you." In this warm atmosphere, it becomes easier for parents to say, "We believe in ourselves!"

If you are already a parent, then your bonds with your new child will be strengthened by your day-by-day confidence in yourself and the good things you are doing. If you are looking forward to a Cesarean birth, then be assured that no matter whether you nurse the baby at birth or only become aware of her existence after many hours, your bonds with your baby are very strong.

> She seemed like a stranger at first. But I got to know what she wanted. In fact, I realized after a few weeks that I could tell what kind of cry it was—hungry, tired, or just plain exasperated. That seemed like a miracle to me. She couldn't even talk, yet we communicated so well. I sat down and wrote a letter to my mother, the first letter in years. I had been depending on the phone, but this seemed so important that I wanted to put it in writing. I wanted to tell her that I was beginning to understand what it means to be a mother, and I wanted to thank her for everything she did for me by raising me.

# TWELVE

# When Something Goes Wrong

Almost all of us, at some time during pregnancy, worry about something going wrong. That's a normal part of adjusting to parenthood. Yet at the very moment we worry, we also don't believe that it will happen to us. We have heard about prematurity, birth defects, and babies who die. But those are unthinkable events that happen to other people.

> When I was in my eighth month, we saw a bad car accident. It made me think about an old wives' tale that unborn babies are affected by things like that. I told my husband what I was thinking, and he just said not to be silly. It did seem silly, so I just tried to put it out of my head. Another time, there was a TV show about birth defects. I turned it off and got busy sorting the baby clothes. . . .

For a few of us, the unthinkable becomes reality. Between 5 and 15 per cent of all pregnancies result in premature babies. Every year, 245,000 babies are born who are classified as premature or having a low birth weight. These days, many babies weighing as little as two pounds at birth survive and live a normal life.

But for premature babies, the first few days or weeks of life are hardly "normal," since both their needs and the care they receive are different from those of a full-term baby. Under these circumstances, the first few weeks of parenthood are not normal either, at least compared to what the parents were expecting.

Perhaps the absence of a gentle phrase to describe "birth defects" is indicative of how uncomfortable the general society feels about these problems. Yet the fact remains that more than 250,000 babies are born with birth defects each year. These can be less significant and easily correctable problems, such as having an extra finger, or major difficulties such as severe heart malformations. By far the majority of birth defects falls somewhere in between. Nonetheless, they can cause significant stress for the child and his family during some or all of his life. Corrective and supportive measures are needed to help the child develop and lead a productive life.

> As soon as the baby started to walk, I noticed that her leg seemed turned and she limped a little. The doctor looked at it and said she would have to wear a cast to fix it. He said she had been born with it. I felt so bad for not noticing sooner, and I worried if there was something else I had missed.

Finally, in this day of modern obstetrics, many babies each year are stillborn or die within the first year after birth. In fact, the United States has a very high rate of infant death. In 1977, the United States ranked seventeenth in the world, far behind such countries as Canada, the Netherlands, and Sweden.

Why bother with such a frightening topic in a book that is meant to be helpful and reassuring about Cesarean birth? It is true that most babies born by Cesarean are completely healthy and normal. But if we look at all the births that do have an unexpected outcome such as prematurity, birth defects, or infant death, then we find that a large percentage of these troubled births are Cesareans. The reason so many of these births are Cesareans is that babies who already have some problem that threatens their well-being might be jeopardized even more by a vaginal birth. In turn, this means that many of the parents who are trying to cope with an unexpected outcome are also trying to recover from a Cesarean birth at the same time. Those of us who "merely" have had a Cesarean know how hard that recovery can be. When recovery is compounded by an unexpected outcome of birth, the result can be temporarily devastating.

They said Jason had a cleft lip, and the pediatrician was leaning over me trying to explain it. I remember he said it wasn't a big problem but that he would have to have surgery. Well, I had just had surgery too for the Cesarean, and they were stitching me up and it was hard to focus on what he meant. I could hear the baby cry and he sounded strong and I just had to pray the baby was OK and I would be OK too.

The first reactions of most parents to an unexpected turn of events are shock and dismay. When something unexpected occurs, you find yourself thinking, "This isn't happening, this can't be happening to me." You wonder if someone hasn't made some mistake.

Often this feeling—"It can't be true"—comes back over and over again. You know what is happening to you and around you, and it is beginning to sink in, but still there are moments when you feel that you're dreaming and you'll wake up any time now.

Another common reaction is guilt. Especially in these days when we know more about good prenatal care, prospective parents can fall into some serious traps. One is to think that only perfection on their part will produce a healthy baby. The other is to think that when they do everything right, a healthy baby is guaranteed. Of course, perfection is impossible. And childbirth is often accompanied by arbitrary developments that have no relationship to how hard the parents or the obstetrician worked to make this into the perfect birth.

I didn't really want this baby at first. We hadn't even been married a year yet, and we had so many plans for just the two of us. When they told me she had breathing problems, I thought, "If she dies, it will be my fault." I felt so miserable that I wanted to die too. I was just sure God was punishing me for thinking all those selfish thoughts when I first got pregnant.

Mixed in with the feelings of unreality and guilt there may be periods of intense anger and frustration. Sometimes you will be able to pinpoint the reason for your anger, as when a neighbor calls who is just plain nosy. At other times, you may feel furious and not have the faintest idea why. It is important to recognize when you are feeling angry. Just saying the words "I'm angry!" to yourself may provide some relief, especially if you remind yourself that this is a normal and legitimate way to feel. Expressing your anger to those around you is also important, but you will find that many people do not really understand what you are going through or how you feel. Once you yourself have identified your feelings, it will be easier for you to exercise some control over how you express them, rather than yielding to the temptation to blow off steam at any handy target.

Along with, or following the anger and guilt, there comes some measure of sadness. This may be a mild kind of transient sadness that results from having to give up a hoped-for experience. For instance, perhaps the parents looked forward to rooming-in and sharing their first few days as a family. Instead, the baby must spend the first few weeks of her life in the neonatal intensive care nursery. Or perhaps the sadness is felt when the parents leave the hospital with empty arms, because their baby requires a longer hospital stay. Another kind of sadness results from having to accept the reality of the baby who has been born, as opposed to the perfection of the baby who was dreamed about.

> My mother always told us what beautiful babies we were, with lots of hair. Well, Rebecca was four weeks early, and the fact that she was bald was really the least of her problems. But when I finally cried, that is what I cried about. I wanted her to be a beautiful baby that everyone oohed and aahed about.

The profound sadness that grieving parents feel when a baby dies is so intense that it is discussed separately, later in this chapter.

Finally, at some point, which may be only days, or which can be years later, there comes the phase of acceptance. This is the stage at which the parents can say, "What happened is not what we wanted, but it *is* what happened. Now we are done with wishing it were different, finding someone to blame, feeling guilty. Now we are ready to move on."

It is very important for parents to realize that their partner probably will not react the same way they do. There is no single correct way to respond when something goes wrong. Each parent will experience the feelings we have described, but seldom to the same degree or at the same time. Nor will each parent express his or her feelings in the identical way. This makes it likely that at any point one of you may feel all alone, perhaps even misunderstood.

> After the baby finally could come home we started having these fights. Usually it would start when I was trying to feed her, and one of the other kids would ask for something or start whining. I would yell at them, and Jack would yell at me for sounding that way. He would say I favored the baby and ignored the other kids and him. I was so tired, I just shut my ears. To be honest, I resented him and the kids for demanding so much. I just wanted to be near the baby and be sure she was still OK.

There is no magic solution for parents when something goes wrong. But it helps—in fact, it is essential—for parents to share their feelings with each other. "Sharing feelings" is almost a cliché, yet it can be the hardest thing in the world to do. You may not want to burden your mate. You may fear that if you start crying, then he will, and then there will be two people feeling miserable instead of just one. You may think that your partner feels so upset that you have to be strong and reassuring for her sake. You may worry that some of your feelings are not normal or rational. But be assured that there is a very wide range of normal responses to unexpected events.

## PREMATURITY AND BIRTH DEFECTS

Having a baby who is premature can be very different from having a baby with a birth defect. From the standpoint of "medical management," however, these two crises may be handled in much the same way. In either situation, parents often are faced with separation from their baby and must absorb and understand some complicated facts about their baby's special problems. In addition, both parents face some challenges to their feelings about themselves.

Even as the babies grow, the similarities are as apparent as the differences. Most premature babies gradually catch up to full-term babies in all respects. Although the premature babies may walk a little later, they get into just as much mischief. By the time they have reached age two, most developmental lags that they had when compared to full-term babies of the same chronological age have disappeared. Similarly, babies whose birth defects are corrected early in life may grow up in such a way that their former defect is genuinely irrelevant to their development.

On the other hand, the effects of severe prematurity and serious birth defects can be lifelong. For families of these children, coping with the stresses of birth and the neonatal period may be the prelude to a lifelong series of adjustments.

### What Is Going On Here? Getting Information When Something Goes Wrong

If your Cesarean was done with a regional anesthetic, you probably suspected or knew from the moment the baby was born that there was some problem. If you had a general anesthetic, your doctor or your husband waited until they thought you were awake enough to accept the information. In either case, you may be as upset by the lack of information as you are by its presence. The baby has some breathing problems, the doctor may say, but we are hopeful that she will be out of the woods entirely within a few days. Right away, you realize that there are no guarantees. Or perhaps you are told that the baby has a cleft lip. She will need surgery, starting soon. But the number and extent of the operations will depend on the success of each previous one, and no one knows with certainty how the baby will look or how much her eating will be interfered with.

In the first few days after the baby's birth, there is another limitation, and that is how much information you can usefully absorb. If the baby's problems are potentially serious, you may lose track of the fact that you are recovering from major surgery. But you are, and your ability to concentrate and to remember what is said to you may be quite limited. It helps to have your husband or some other person with you when you are talking to the doctor. The two of you together will do a much better job of remembering what is said. Just the fact that both of you are hearing the same words will help to reduce confusion and misunderstanding. Be sure to ask all the questions you think of. And don't hesitate to ask the same questions more than once so that you can feel sure you understand what is going on.

In general, you need three kinds of information. The first type is, "What are the baby's problems?" Next comes, "What is being done to help with these problems, and what risks are associated with these treatments?" Finally there is, "What do you expect the results of the baby's treatment to be?"

Some doctors don't like to give much information. They may think that you won't understand, or they may think that they are helping by not scaring you. But there are ways to translate medical facts into nonmedical people's language. You will probably imagine things that are far worse than the truth. So let the doctor know that you want to talk regularly, several times a day, if the situation is unstable and changing hour by hour.

Some doctors feel that they owe it to their patients to be totally honest, which to them means emphasizing the worst possible outcome for the baby. The theory behind this is that if the baby does die, you will have been prepared, and if she doesn't, no harm was done. However, we are learning that a lot of harm may be done when doctors discourage parents from having hope. Certainly, if your baby is expected to die, you should be told. But most babies who are premature or have a birth defect do not die. Yet parents who are discouraged from having hope begin "anticipatory grieving," preparing for the loss they are told may face them. Unfortunately, it can then be very difficult to reverse the process and begin building close, loving ties with the infant. Even when the baby is declared well enough to come home from the hospital, you may still hear the doctor's early warnings in your mind and feel a distance between yourself and your child.

You deserve all the information you can get. You also deserve to have realistic hopes for the best possible future for you and your baby. You may have to insist that you get the information and support you need.

### Separation: Did I Really Have a Baby?

Most of the time, babies who are premature or who have a birth defect are separated from their parents for at least a little while. In fact, Cesarean babies with no problems at all are routinely kept in the intensive care nursery for a twenty-four hour period of observation in many hospitals. So when the infant does have a problem, the separation may stretch out to many days. The Cesarean mother who cannot see and care for her baby immediately has nothing but her own discomfort and her own worst fears to concentrate on.

A new trend in neonatal care has led to the establishment of regional intensive care units for infants. This means that if your baby's problems would be better cared for in a specialized facility, she may be moved to a hospital miles from where you are. It is bad enough to have your baby down the hall in the nursery when you cannot get around on your own. But mother and baby being in different hospitals can be very stressful for both parents. The father may be visiting his wife, traveling many miles to visit the baby, and even trying to care for children at home as well. The mother, meanwhile, is trying to put together a hasty recovery so she can be discharged and begin visiting her baby. Yet she may be frantic with worry, and this surely does not contribute to a rapid recovery from her Cesarean. So, although these regional units make the most advanced care available to babies who need it, they can create tremendous problems for the family.

> I didn't have a moment to stop and think. I was either with my wife or the baby every waking moment. In a situation where nothing was going very well, it helped me to stay so busy.

Whether your separation from the baby is forty feet or forty miles, and whether it is one day or seven, there are some things you can do to help yourself get through it. One is to ask the nurses or your husband to take pictures of your baby. Even if the baby is receiving special care and seems to have tubes and wires everywhere, she is your baby, and pictures can really help you during the period of separation.

While you are separated, you also need another kind of information from the medical facts mentioned earlier. Although you cannot care for the baby, you should be aware of the kind of routine care being given, as this will help to give you a sense of your baby's reality. You can ask your husband or one of the nurses on the floor to help you here. They can give you regular reports on simple things, whether the baby is awake or asleep, being changed or being fed, opening her eyes, responding to stimulation. These are the things that you would notice if you could be there, and although it is a bittersweet happiness to hear about them second-hand, it does help. Do not worry about bothering the nurses. They know that you are concerned and want to keep in close touch. If they are too busy to answer your questions, ask them to suggest a better time for you to call. There may be one nurse on each shift who is responsible for your baby's care. If not, you may find it helpful to get to know a particular nurse on each of the shifts and then ask for her each time you call. Some regional intensive care centers now have special free hotlines that make it possible for parents to call the floor twenty-four hours a day to ask how or what their baby is doing.

Occasionally, hospitals have made arrangements for mothers and babies to be transported together if the baby must be moved to a regional intensive care unit. This new practice is not observed in most areas, and the fact that you have had a Cesarean birth will make your transfer an even more complicated undertaking. It is not considered good medical practice to transfer the postoperative care of a patient (even if she is a mother) from one doctor and facility to another doctor and facility, unless there is some medical reason that justifies such a transfer. In addition, although you gain closeness to your baby by being transferred, you may lose closeness to your own obstetrician and hospital, and your other family members. If you are convinced that this alternative is best for you and your family, you should ask your doctor about it. If he or she refuses, be sure you understand what the medical reasons are. If you are doing well, then your very early discharge may be an acceptable solution.

In situations where the baby's problems can be anticipated, some doctors are now following a policy of transferring pregnant mothers to the hospital with the regional neonatal intensive care unit just before the baby is born. This "transfer" of the baby before birth is probably safer for the baby, as well as having the advantage of avoiding prolonged separation. Such a transfer often means changing doctors.

### Feeding the Baby

While you were pregnant, you undoubtedly gave a lot of thought to how to feed the baby. If you decided to use formula, then your Cesarean birth and the baby's problems at birth will not affect your plans. But if you had plans to breast-feed your baby, you may feel discouraged and wonder if your plans must be changed. There are a few birth defects that preclude breast-feeding. But these are rare, and most mothers who want to breast-feed their baby can do so in spite of surgical birth and prematurity or birth defect. It does require extra support and patience, but the rewards are tremendous.

We now know that breast milk provides immunological benefits that formula does not. For the baby with problems at birth, this can be even more beneficial. And if you manage to breast-feed your baby in spite of the obstacles, you will find that your own self-esteem increases rapidly. You may have needed your doctor's help in delivering the baby and you may depend on the nurses to care for the baby now, but you can still provide breast milk! (Please see Chapter Seven, "Your Baby's First Week of Life," for helpful hints on breast-feeding.)

It will be necessary to pump your breasts if you and the baby are in separate hospitals, or if you return home before the baby can be released. Expressing breast milk is not something that just comes naturally to all of us, so don't hesitate to ask for help. The nurses or your La Leche League members can supply a breast pump and also offer the practical tips and emotional support that you will need at this time.

The best things you can do for yourself may also be the hardest, and those are to rest and take care of yourself. Your baby is in good hands, and your breast milk is a way of getting you two together even before you can begin full-time motherhood.

### The First Visit: How Can I Love This Baby? How Can I Not Love This Baby?

At some point, which may come soon or seem like forever, you will be able to see your baby. Since no parent has a perfect baby, all of us are faced with the job of reconciling the real baby we have created with the ideal we had dreamed of. But the baby who is premature or has a birth defect poses special problems for her parents in this respect. Premature babies have scrawny limbs, and their heads look big by comparison to the rest of their bodies. Their movements often seem jerky, and their breathing is commonly irregular or seems labored. The child with a birth defect may also have special problems relating to her physical appearance, depending on the type of birth defect she has. In preparation for the first visit, it may help to have your husband or one of the nurses explain in advance what you will see.

If your baby does need special care, she may seem to have wires and tubes attached to every conceivable spot. This can be very frightening, to say the least. All the equipment, the machines, they all seem so foreign, and the baby looks so small and helpless.

There you are, barely recovering from your surgery, and trying to adjust to the shock of seeing the baby, perhaps for the first time. You may find that your love and concern are all mixed up with apprehension and a sense of alienation from this frail infant. Some mothers in this situation even feel a strong impulse to run away. They doubt that they can love this baby—they may even feel repulsed—and they worry that they will not be able to care for the baby properly.

Even mothers who fall in love with the baby at first sight may feel helpless at this first visit. You weren't prepared for the baby to have problems, and you don't know how to act now. Can you touch the baby? You certainly don't want to do anything that won't be good for her or that will interfere with nursery routines.

Fortunately, there is a lot you can do for your baby. It may take a while for you to feel comfortable doing it, but you have an essential role to play in her growth and development. As soon as you feel able and as soon as the nursery's policies will let you, get going on parenthood! You may change the diaper of even the tiniest baby. You may nurse the baby or help with feedings if she is a little bigger and the feedings are going well. The amazing thing is that simply touching your baby can make a major contribution to improving her condition. Research shows that premature babies who receive this extra attention from parents or parent substitutes have improved breathing, are more relaxed, gain weight more rapidly, and have better physical development. And, of course, when you get involved with your baby's care, it helps you to get past that first-visit shaky feeling and really get to know your baby for the individual she is.

### As Time Goes On

The rules and practices of intensive care nurseries vary around the country. Once, parents were allowed to view their infants through a glass panel during limited "visiting" hours. Now many nurseries not only allow parents to come in, they also encourage them to come. Depending on your baby's condition at birth, you may have a very limited role in her care at the beginning, or you may quickly assume as much of her care as your own condition permits. Regardless of how long or how short the baby's period of special care is, there are some practical tips that you can keep in mind to help you get through this time.

1. *Visit your baby often.* If you and the baby are in the same hospital, your visits will still have to be limited by your own physical recovery from the Cesarean. But babies who are prema-

ture or need special care often sleep much more than full-term babies. You may need to spend hours in the nursery just to enjoy the few moments when the baby's eyes are open and she can respond to you. Ask the nurses if the baby's condition permits waking her. If she is under special lights and must have eye patches, ask if the lights can be turned off and the patches removed while you are visiting so that the baby can see you.

If you have been discharged while the baby remains hospitalized, that long trek to see the baby may seem discouraging. You wonder if it really matters to the baby that you are there. It almost seems as though the baby belongs to the nurses, not to you. It is harder for you, as the parent of a child with special needs, to feel close to your baby. This is partly because you don't get as much encouragement or feedback from your baby as other parents do. So you may have to push yourself to keep visiting, and you are likely to feel depressed and discouraged about yourself as a parent. But you are important to that baby. Try to visit once each day during the early part of your own recovery, if distances will permit it. Do not push yourself to do more than you are physically capable of handling, which is very little. The time will come when you can assume full responsibility for your baby's care.

2. *Take care of yourself.* This is not the time to pull a Superwoman routine. Rest often. Get friends or relatives to help with other children or to bring in meals. When someone says, "Is there anything I can do to help?" say, "Yes!" and then let them know what your needs are. After all, if the roles were reversed, you would be eager to help your friends. Even if you are well on the road to recovery and your baby is making terrific progress, this is still a time of tremendous stress for you and for everyone close to you. Try to keep life as simple as possible. Do only what is absolutely necessary and important to you, and let the rest wait.

3. *Talk to each other.* It's easy to get into the routine of taking turns being with the baby while your mate stays at home, sleeps, or goes to work. Like ships passing in the night, you are aware of each other's presence, but your paths hardly cross. This leaves you wide open for problems between you. It is essential that you

find regular times to sit down together without interruption. Use the times to talk about the baby, yourselves, whatever seems to be on your mind at the time.

> I worried about Caroline for what seemed like days. I knew she was exhausted, and so was I, and I thought I probably should be doing more. When we finally had some time together, it turned out that she had the same worries about herself, that she should be doing more to support me.

4. *Name your baby.* Some parents of premature babies or those with birth defects delay naming their baby. Probably it has something to do with feeling distant from the baby, and also with the parents' fears about whether the baby will survive. Experience now shows that no matter what happens, you will be able to deal with it better if you give your baby the identity of having her own name.

5. *Ask questions.* Don't worry about sounding silly or bothering the staff. Their job will be much easier if you have the information and support you need. This is all very new to you, and the very unfamiliarity of it makes your adjustment more difficult. Getting your questions answered in words you can understand is an important way of coping with what is happening.

### Becoming a Family

When a baby is born, a family is born too. But the baby who is premature or has special needs may seem unreal, removed, living in her plastic-covered isolette. Parents often express the feeling that the baby "isn't really mine" until she can come out of the isolette or until she can come home. In order to help parents make that transition to the day when the baby is really theirs, some hospitals now make arrangements for the mother to re-enter the hospital for two or three days before the baby is released, so that she may take over the full care of the baby in the hospital.

> I cried when they said she could come home. Even though it had been only three weeks, I felt so empty and worried. Finally, I thought, finally I'm going to be a mother.

Along with the joys of having your baby at home at last, there may come some lingering worries. Can I really be a good parent? Will the baby gain weight as quickly at home as she did in the hospital? Hopefully you will be in touch with a pediatrician, pediatric nurse practitioner, or family doctor who will understand your normal need for continuing reassurance and support.

Parents worry about the long-range future too. Will my baby who was premature always be fragile? Will my baby with a cleft lip be stared at or teased as an older child? It may be helpful to remind yourself that some of the most brilliant people in history have been premature or had a birth defect. The label itself does not necessarily mean anything—bad or good—about your child's future.

Some parents worry about whether their child may have suffered brain damage that is yet undetected. It is true that some kinds of brain damage are not uncovered in infancy. But the reverse is also true: Infants who are thought to have suffered brain damage often turn out to be perfectly normal and healthy. In one hospital, doctors examined all the premature and full-term babies who were suspected of having brain damage. Even though the doctors used every tool available to measure the babies' neurological condition, only 50 per cent of the infants were given a diagnosis that later proved correct. At this early stage, only the most severe brain damage can accurately be identified by your doctor, and in that case it is likely that you will also be able to identify the signs that the baby has suffered brain damage.

If you asked your doctor about brain damage and the answer was that he or she didn't know, your doctor was being truthful. If he or she answered that your baby does not have brain damage, then your doctor was using past experience as a foundation for this judgment. He or she was saying, in effect, "Babies who are born under these circumstances seldom suffer brain damage." Your doctor was also saying something very essential to you as a parent, and that is that vague, global fears that you may have about your baby can interfere with your abilities as a parent. Realistically, we know that some babies with markedly low birth weights or serious birth defects have more than their share of problems in later years. But this does not mean that your baby will have these problems. And worrying about something before it is even a reality can be damaging to your baby and to you.

If your baby does not have any enduring problems, the best therapy for you is time. You will get to know this new individual, and in the process you will learn new things about yourself as well. You will make mistakes as a parent, as all of us do. Your baby will get diaper rash and have sleepless nights. And you will relax and realize that these problems are a normal part of parenting, not connected at all with how the baby got her start. In fact, it may seem good to settle down to just everyday problems.

If your baby is one of those whose special needs continue, then your lives will be irrevocably changed. The stresses on families for whom doctors' offices and hospitals become second homes are enormous. There are studies that show that families of a child with serious birth defects are more vulnerable to severe marital and family problems. The best insurance against such problems is to join a parents' group or get involved in supportive counseling from a professional. There are self-help parent support groups springing up all over the country, and the need for them grows as more children who previously might not have survived birth are saved. If you cannot find such a group in your area, perhaps your doctor or childbirth instructor will help you start one. The people who can help you the most are other parents who really understand what you are going through, because they have been through it themselves.

### Feelings About Yourself

Probably all parents use their children as one yardstick to measure themselves. We say that a baby "has his mother's eyes," or seems very active, "like his father." In fact, a newborn hardly has an identity of her own, since she is only recently separated from her mother's body. How, then, do you explain that a baby is premature or has a birth defect? Whose "fault" is it? What kind of parents are you who produced this child?

These seem like terribly harsh questions. But they are the kinds of questions that parents ask all the time, either aloud or to themselves. Did I do something wrong? Why wasn't the baby born in the "normal" way and at the "normal" time? Why isn't this baby like all the others?

To begin with, it is essential to do this soul-searching out loud. If there is some identifiable cause of your baby's problem, then you should know about it. More than likely, however, the doctor will answer that the cause is unknown. More than half of the premature births cannot be explained. (The remainder are caused mostly by certain medical conditions in the mother. Some of these, such as diabetes, lead to an intentionally premature birth because at this time it carries fewer risks than allowing the pregnancy to go to full term.) Similarly, the causes of birth defects are not understood in the great majority of cases. Current theory is that some combination of heredity and environment causes most birth defects.

Once you have determined the facts that are known, you will probably have many feelings about yourself left to deal with. If the doctor can't explain what happened, you may be tempted to "fill in the blank" with guilt, anger, or just a sense of inadequacy and failure. If this baby is your measuring stick, you feel that you don't measure up.

There are a number of reasons why parents feel this way, and understanding these reasons will help you to deal with your feelings. First, let's not lose track of some basic facts about you. Like all new parents, you are dealing with the physiological changes of the postpartum period. This means that you are on an emotional roller coaster, and nothing but time can end the ride. Second, you are recovering from major abdominal surgery. Many women feel inadequate just because they did not have a vaginal birth, and you are coping with far more stress than they are. So you are entitled to feel upset or blue. In fact, it is almost inevitable. And just as inevitably, you will recover your strength and your good feelings about yourself.

In addition to coping with the physical changes that are occurring, you will have to deal with the question, "Why me?" This is a question that almost all parents ask when their baby is premature or has a birth defect. In searching for an answer, they may fasten on something that has no relationship whatever to the outcome of the pregnancy.

> All through my pregnancy, my mother made comments about the fact that I wanted to work up to the end. Sometimes it seemed like she was paying me a compliment, like when she said she would never have had that much energy, but there was always an edge of criticism or worry in her voice. When my labor started three weeks before my due date, my first thought was, "Mom was right; now look what I've done."

It is essential for parents to talk to each other and to talk to the doctor about these troublesome fears. Hearing that you are not to blame may be enough to reassure you. Some parents want to have the additional reassurance of reading about the particular problem their baby has.

Sometimes there is a relationship between some trait of the mother or father and its effects on the baby, as in the case of maternal diabetes. Yet it is not the mother's fault if she is diabetic or Rh negative. It is not the father's fault if he carries some recessive genes that combined with his wife's genes and some environmental factors, result in a birth defect. Nor is it the doctor's fault.

When the cause is unclear, parents may search their minds and hearts to see if they have somehow done something to deserve this. And, since no one is perfect, they may well come up with something from their past about which they feel guilty and for which they may think they are being punished. Although this is not a theology book, we want to emphasize that few religions or philosophies would support the notion that parents are being punished by having a baby who is premature or has a birth defect. In fact, all full-term, healthy babies are born to imperfect parents! You do not "deserve" your baby's condition, but it is a reality. In the final analysis, only you can come to terms with the question, "Why me?" Once you find an answer, or accept the fact that there may be no answer, then you will be a happier person and a better parent.

## WHEN THE BABY DIES

Most couples of childbearing age don't have much experience with death. Even if you have coped with the loss of a parent or loved one, there is nothing that can prepare you for the crushing grief that comes when a baby dies at birth or soon after.

In this section, we want to reach out to those of you whose babies have died. Unlike other portions of this book, we have not filled these pages with reassuring words and upbeat suggestions for making life better. Nothing can take away your loss. But we can give you some information about what has helped other couples. We hope that it will help you as you grieve, and as you find the strength to go on.

It is difficult to describe the feelings of parents when a baby dies. In the first day or two, you are quite literally in shock. You may be unable to hear the doctor's words, or you may try to convince yourself that it just isn't true.

The nurse left and got the doctor and he couldn't find the heartbeat either. I just refused to believe it. They gave me the spinal, and then the baby was born. Then they let Dick in and said, "Do you want to hold her?" and then I believed it. Dick held her and I touched her tiny fingers and her toes and cried and cried. I never stopped crying even after they took her away and finished stitching me up.

Often, everything feels very jumbled and confusing in those first days. There are strange new decisions that seem very difficult. The hospital may want to know what the baby's name is, even if she is stillborn. And what will you do with the baby's body? The hospital will make arrangements if you wish, but first they will give you the opportunity to contact a funeral director and arrange matters yourself. Should there be a funeral? If so, who should be there and what should be said? Informal observations by professionals tend to indicate that having a funeral service helps to make the baby's birth and death more real, which in turn helps parents to deal with what happened. On the other hand, the parents' personal beliefs are the best guidelines for how to proceed.

Your doctor will ask for your permission to perform an autopsy. Again, your personal or religious beliefs should be your guides. If having an autopsy is congruent with your beliefs, then it is a good idea to go ahead. Although many of these examinations are inconclusive, you will have the satisfaction of knowing that every attempt has been made to come to some scientific understanding of why your baby died. And if there is concrete evidence to explain the baby's death, it will make your adjustment slightly easier.

You need help and support from every quarter at this time. Your husband or a relative may be permitted to stay with you while you are still hospitalized. You and your family should be sure to arrange things so that there is still someone with you for the first two to four weeks at home. Aside from your family, your clergyman can be an invaluable source of support, even if you haven't been to a service in years. Most hospitals have pastoral counselors and/or social workers who will feel comfortable with and be supportive to you.

The head nurse came in to talk to me the day after the baby died. She seemed so uncomfortable, and I think she was there just because she thought it was her duty. She said a few things that were meant to make me feel better. When she said, "I suppose you had the nursery all ready and everything," I started to bawl again. She looked kind of scared and said, "You need someone to talk to," and half an hour later the social worker came in. She turned out to be the most understanding and helpful person. She stayed for almost two hours and came back the next day too.

When you are in the midst of such tremendous emotional turmoil it is hard to be aware of other things going on simultaneously. It may be helpful, then, as you mourn your child, to remind yourself of the enormous physiological strains that are occurring during this early grieving period. You are recovering from major abdominal surgery. Because of this, your energy is terribly limited. Eventually, you will want to get moving, to begin going out in the world again. Yet even months after the birth, you may still feel some effects from your surgery.

In addition, as cruel and ironic as it seems, you are enduring the tremendous physical changes that every mother experiences at the end of a pregnancy, even though your baby has died. You may have wild mood swings, unlike any you have ever felt before. These are due, at least in part, to the hormonal changes going on inside you.

There used to be an injection that was routinely given to women who were not breast-feeding, in order to help dry up their milk. It has now been determined that its value was greatly over-rated and it may cause some side effects, so many doctors and hospitals have stopped using it. Those who do use the injection now often give their patients a written statement describing the possible dangers. Thus, another cruel irony is that most women whose babies die must endure the period when their milk comes in and slowly dries up. Women who have had Cesareans experience the hardest part of this adjustment while still hospitalized. Some hospitals use binders to help with this problem, although there appears to be an increased incidence of blocked ducts and infection with their use. Ice packs help some women, while the application of heat helps others. Like the loss of the baby, this is something that mostly must be endured because there is no other way.

## The First Few Weeks at Home

Very few parents feel able to resume their usual activities during this time. Although the father may return to work, perhaps part-time at first, couples seldom wish to go out or see any but their closest friends. Both parents feel such sadness and suffering, and their tears may be touched off by the slightest reminder of the baby or the plans they had. Many parents, especially mothers, have trouble sleeping. Naps during the day can help, but often no amount of sleep feels restful. There is some comfort in resuming normal routines, yet getting through each day takes all your strength.

Again, many unfamiliar and troublesome questions arise: What shall we do with the baby's things, her room, her furniture? No matter what the decision is, it should be the parents' decision. Well-meaning relatives or friends who want to whisk away all of the reminders of the baby are making a mistake. If this has happened to you, you may want to consider taking out the baby's things and re-storing them in your own time and in your own way. And, no matter how the baby's belongings are put away, there may be times when you wish to take them out again and look at them. This is not a morbid wish, and you should certainly do it if you want to, even if it makes you cry.

What shall we tell other people? In the early weeks, an obituary is helpful. You may want to enlist trusted friends or relatives to help you inform people. This can be accomplished by asking one person in each setting where you are known—work, neighborhood, church—to be responsible for telling everyone in that setting.

How can people help? Many will want to send flowers or do something to make a concrete demonstration of their sympathy. If flowers seem out of place to you after the first few bouquets, you may want to consider establishing a memorial fund. It is not necessary to decide immediately what to do with the money. Simply designate someone (perhaps your clergyman) to receive the funds for the (baby's name) Memorial Fund, and then you can decide where to donate the money at a later time. Or, if you want a more immediate and practical approach, just ask your friends to send over a casserole. You will not feel up to organizing and cooking a meal for quite a long time.

These are some of the concrete issues that grieving parents face. But overriding all of the practical problems are your feelings at this time. Again, because we have not endured or been exposed to such grief before, few of us recognize the normal aspects of grieving.

You may have strong feelings of unreality. You seem to be walking in a dream, a nightmare. It is very difficult to focus on anything or concentrate on what is being said to you. You have difficulty remembering things. The simplest tasks take on enormous proportions. Getting washed and choosing clothes to wear that day may seem to use up all your strength.

Many grieving parents, women in particular, report having periods of panic or strange physical sensations. This can be so unusual that you start to worry that you may be going crazy. Your doctor can help you separate those physical sensations, which are caused by grieving, from any that might need medical attention. Parents also commonly report being preoccupied with the baby and feeling moments of intense longing. These may be coupled with brief seconds of "forgetting" that the baby has died and imagining that she is crying, or that they will see her soon.

During the mourning process, parents often go over and over their pregnancy for any evidence that they contributed to the death of their child. Since none of us is perfect, they probably can find something to feel guilty about. One mother said, "I took all those heartburn tablets and never asked my doctor." Another blamed a medication that her doctor had prescribed, and declared that she was sure it would be found to cause stillbirths in the years to come, even though there was absolutely no evidence to support her idea. A husband confessed that he had had a brief affair years before, and wondered if he was being punished in some way for his infidelity. If there has been an autopsy, the results may help you to put some of your guilt aside. Again, however, in infant deaths where there was no prior warning that something was wrong, the autopsy results are commonly inconclusive. You may have to be the one to convince yourself that you did not cause your baby's death. You can do that if you ask for all of the information that is available to the doctor about what happened, and if you share your guilty worries with your husband or your doctor, and if you give yourself enough time. You did not "deserve" to have your baby die.

Because you have suffered such a loss, such a tremendously unfair blow, you may also find yourself feeling very angry. Your well-meaning friends may seem too interfering, or completely without any real understanding of what you are going through.

You may get angry at each other, God, the doctor, or the TV, which insists on showing rosy-bottomed babies in disposable diaper ads. Those around you who reach out in sympathy and catch your anger instead may back off.

> When Sharon finally came to visit me, she seemed uncomfortable. We talked about everything but the baby. She chattered on and on about work until I thought I would scream. I had thought she was a good friend, but when she left I thought I never wanted to see her again.

In fact, you may feel such a strong sense of alienation from friends that you don't care what you say to them or how they feel about it. This, too, is normal, and the best friends are patient and allow you to use their help and support in your own way and time.

Unfortunately, in this country, there are not even any reliable traditions to fall back on when a baby dies. Some people find that they cannot tolerate the idea of an infant's death, and so they make excuses and avoid contacting you. If this happens to you, no doubt you will feel hurt. Later on, when your wounds have healed, you can stop to recognize that it was your friends' pain, not their uncaring, that prevented them from reaching out to you.

> The craziest thing was that I felt I had to take care of everyone else. My baby was dead, and yet people did not know what to say or how to act around me, and I ended up taking the lead and bringing it up and letting them know that I was getting better.

### Telling Your Other Children

If this was not your first baby, it is essential that you discuss the baby's death with your other children. The main points to remember are to keep your explanations simple, but to share your feelings freely. Don't blame God for the baby's death, because your children will have mixed feelings about God if you do. Don't pretend to be cheerful for your children's sake, although there will certainly be moments when you feel deep consolation in their presence. Explain to the children that the baby died, and describe the cause in the simplest terms if it is known. Allow your children to ask their own questions, rather than giving them more information than they can understand or are ready to hear. It also helps, if you are a religious person, to say that the baby has "gone to be with God," or whatever simple words describe your beliefs. Do not say that the baby has gone to sleep, as this may make younger children fearful of falling asleep themselves. Don't be surprised if children under the age of five do not understand the concept of forever, and keep expecting that the baby will stop being dead. Older children may wish to attend the baby's funeral if you have one, and this is often helpful for them in dealing with the reality of the situation.

At first, it may be very difficult to include your children in your grieving. You may want to be alone, and feel unable to answer even their simplest questions. As soon as you are up to it, you should spend time with them and start talking about what has happened. The children need to be reassured that you are still alive and still care for them. If you feel unable to be with them, let them know that your crying and being alone will help you to feel better, and that you will be able to play with them and care for them completely again as time goes by. Make sure that whoever is helping you understands how to talk to the children about the baby's death and about your needs.

Later on, as you begin to resume your normal routine, there will still be many times when you remember the baby and when the tears begin again. Share these times with your children, and let them cry with you if they want to. Even the smallest child will want to console you and be consoled by you. Children's worst fears about death arise when it is treated as a terrible secret and when adults attempt to hide it or disguise their feelings about it.

### My Spouse Doesn't Understand

There is no single "right" way to grieve the loss of a baby. Furthermore, parents often do not move through the stages of grieving at the same time or with the same intensity. It is also true that, in the case of infant death, the tremendous physical impact of the experience is all reserved for the mother. She has felt the baby's life within her, she has given birth. She has, in effect, lost a part of herself when the baby dies. Thus it is almost always true that mothers respond more intensely to a baby's death, and their grief is much more debilitating for a longer period of time. Unfortunately, this creates a situation ripe for conflict between the parents.

> I couldn't understand how he could laugh so hard at a stupid TV show just two weeks after she died. I felt like he had just forgotten her completely, like he was wiping her memory away so fast, and I wanted to hang onto her memory even more to make it up to her for how he acted.

Sometimes these conflicts will pass and be forgotten. But much too often, they build and escalate beyond the ability of either partner to make them stop. In fact, there is a very high incidence of separation and/or divorce following the death of a child. (Other social disasters, including alcoholism and suicide, are also alarmingly common as the aftermath of such a crisis.)

Some understanding of what is going on here may help you to stay together through this time of extreme stress. It is a common misconception that sharing a disaster brings people closer to each other. Although this may be true in some situations, the reverse is often true when a baby dies. Both parents have suffered a tremendous blow. Each is emotionally depleted, even devastated. Each is vulnerable and needs every ounce of strength to keep going and to strive toward recovery. There is literally no emotional energy left to give to the other. You are stricken and bereft. How can you summon the extra resources required to soothe your partner?

There are also some simple differences of style that can lead to tremendous misunderstandings. Under normal circumstances, you may be able to accept that your spouse is very quiet and a loner, while you are more talkative and gregarious. Yet when you are grief-stricken, your spouse's silence and withdrawal make you feel like you have been abandoned. For his part, he may criticize your talking and seeking the company of friends as unfeeling behavior. This is a time, more than any other, when you need to be tolerant of each other's differences.

If your disagreements and problems with each other cannot be contained, now is the time to get help. Sometimes a few discussions with your doctor may help. By now you will know whether he or she seems to be a sympathetic and helpful person. If you are lucky, there may be professional people in your area with experience in the kind of crisis intervention counseling that grieving couples may need. If not, most counselors can at least help you negotiate a truce. The best help of all may come from a grieving parents' organization, or a death-and-dying self help group. The members of such a group have all experienced the death of a loved one, whether at birth or at a later age. They understand some of what each of you are facing, and they will offer sympathetic and practical advice. Your pediatrician or childbirth education organization should know if there is such a group in your area.

### From Suffering to Acceptance
Gradually, very gradually, your suffering will become less. Though nothing will ever replace your baby, you will find that you can resume some of your former activities. Memories of your pregnancy and the baby's birth and death will not always be accompanied by the stabbing pain that they used to bring. Indeed, you will even be able to enjoy the present and to feel some zest for life.

One of the most painful and most important parts of your recovery will be the "first times" or milestones you must face. Something as simple as seeing your hairdresser for the first time after the baby's death may be terribly painful for you; or the milestone may be an occasion that you had anticipated joyfully during pregnancy, such as a birthday or a holiday, which now must be faced with empty arms. There is a temptation to avoid these milestones because they seem to threaten the little bit of solace or peace that you may have achieved. Yet, painful as they are, facing each milestone makes the next step much easier, and so paves your way back into the world. Though you dread each of your milestones, you may look forward to some relief and renewed strength after you get through each one.

Anniversaries become very important and often painful to

grieving parents. At first you may simply find that you are feeling sadder on the day of the week the baby died, or the day of the week the funeral was held. Gradually, you will notice that it is no longer the day of the week, but the date each month that reminds you of your loss. Eventually you will find that the important anniversaries connected with the baby are reduced to a few occasions each year, usually the anniversary of the baby's death and those holidays that are traditionally joyful family events for you.

Another aspect of recovery that is difficult is the occurrence of what feel like major setbacks, when the grief that you are feeling returns to its former intensity. This may happen at any time, even as long as a year after the baby's death. It does not happen to everyone, but it is a normal part of grieving for some people. If you have such a recurrence, it does not mean that you have lost all of the ground you thought was gained. Again, time will come to your rescue, and the terrible debilitation that you feel will change to normal functioning again.

What does acceptance feel like? When a baby dies, the fact that life goes on around you seems irrelevant, or even like a cruel joke at first. Gradually, the fact that there is life still going on around you becomes a diversion. Occasionally it may even seem interesting. In the end, it is your salvation. When you have reached this phase you will be able to say, "Although I am deeply grieved at the loss of my child, I also feel great joy in the fact that I am alive."

There is no timetable for acceptance. It is seldom achieved before several months have passed, and it is normal for parents to be aware of grieving for years, although certainly not with the same intensity of the early months.

### Having Another Baby

No one can tell you what is best. There are many theories about this issue, but the decision in the end is a personal one. Some couples wish to start another pregnancy immediately. A few decide never to have another baby.

First of all, you must be certain that your physical condition warrants another pregnancy. Although many doctors advocate waiting at least a year before beginning another pregnancy, many women become pregnant much sooner without any problem. Probably the main issue for the grieving couple is this: You cannot replace the baby who died. You can have another baby, but you cannot get this baby back. If you are in a hurry to console yourself for this loss by having another baby, you may never finish grieving for this baby and you may place tremendous burdens on the "replacement" baby. On the other hand, doctors have observed that women whose babies die, especially when it was their first pregnancy, never feel confident about themselves as childbearers until they have delivered a healthy second child. They may be reassured by their doctor's statistics about how unlikely it is for anything to go wrong again, but they never fully believe in themselves until they have their own personal proof.

Three months? Six months? A year or two? There is no firm rule, at least none with any scientific defense. Consult with your husband, your doctor, your heart—you will certainly worry throughout your next pregnancy, no matter what anyone says to reassure you. Do *not* accept anyone's advice that another baby would be good for you, until you feel ready to have another baby.

Some parents find it helpful to have genetic counseling when they begin looking forward to another pregnancy. In all likelihood, your baby's death was not related to any genetic problem. However, when such a tragic event remains unexplained, it may be comforting to parents to know that they have left no stone unturned. If you are interested in genetic counseling, ask your doctor if he or she feels that it is indicated. This kind of counseling is a specialized service not available in every area, and you will want to balance your wish to have such counseling against the time, expense, and possibly travel involved in getting the services of a trained genetic counselor.

# THIRTEEN

# Having Another Cesarean

You are pregnant again, or thinking about getting pregnant. It may not be an easy decision, and sometimes the prospect of another Cesarean delivery does not make it any easier. Even if your first Cesarean was not a bad experience, few women look forward to having surgery. If you are looking forward to your first Cesarean, but you already have children at home, then you have joined a growing minority of childbearing couples. Even women who have successfully delivered vaginally may have a subsequent Cesarean. Whether you are planning a second Cesarean or planning a first when brothers and sisters already exist, the project you have begun is somewhat different from getting ready for a first baby.

When the birth is going to be a "repeat" (second or more) Cesarean, the first step is to sit down and talk over what happened the first time. You will undoubtedly recall events or procedures, but by now the reasons they occurred may seem hazy. In addition, there will be differences that each of you will hope for this time. Some of the differences will be in the area of doctors' and hospitals' policies, such as allowing the father to be present at the birth or permitting sibling visitation during your hospital stay. Others will be based on your awareness that medical circumstances change from one birth to the next.

> Because I was bleeding, they had to put me to sleep. I hated missing out on his birth that way. My doctor knew how I felt, but there was just no other way. This time, I am going to have a spinal. I don't care about anything else, as long as we have a healthy baby and I am awake when it is born.

Unfortunately, Cesarean couples sometimes miss out on some aspect of birth that they would have valued, simply because they did not know what was possible. As you review your previous experience, it will be helpful to do it in the manner of people who are "brainstorming" a problem or an idea. Let your imagination roam freely, and don't stop to worry about what is sensible or realistic, at least not in this stage of your planning. You may wish to consult the list of Family Centered Cesarean Birth options (Chapter Fifteen) in order to stimulate your thinking about how you would like this next birth to be.

Once you have completely reviewed your past experience and simultaneously begun a list for the future, you will want to find out what options and resources are already available to you. Your childbirth preparation group can help you become familiar with the current picture in your area. If it has been a while since your last child was born, you may have some pleasant surprises in store for you. Many doctors and hospitals are changing their policies to better meet the needs of the Cesarean family.

> Somebody told me that all the hospitals have rooming-in now, no matter if it was a Cesarean or not. I know that I would have felt better last time if I could have had the baby more. It was such a relief to know that this time would be different.

This is also a good time to find out if there is a Cesarean parents' support group in your area. This may be an independently organized group, or a committee or task force within your childbirth preparation group. The Cesarean parents' group can provide social and emotional support, plus plenty of practical tips about how to make this birth the best possible experience.

As you talk to each other and to other supportive people, you will begin to develop priorities. For many couples, the biggest priority is something they were unable to have last time, such as being together for the birth. Other couples get a tremendous amount of satisfaction just from planning this birth to the fullest, even if they have to compromise on many of the details of the birth. It makes up for the shock and fear associated with the last time, and gives them back their sense of autonomy.

Once you have started these early stages of the planning, it is time to visit your doctor. You may even discover that you are one of the many women who could deliver vaginally, even though you had one Cesarean. (See Chapter Two.) In any case, his or her help in this stage is essential, since he or she can review the causes and circumstances of your previous Cesarean with you. Sometimes, however, the parts of the birth that couples most treasure or dread are the details that the doctor, who attends hundreds of births each year, may not recall specifically.

If you are clear about what happened to you and what you hope will happen this time, then this is the time to begin preliminary planning discussions with your doctor. Some compromise will certainly be necessary, so it is essential that you remember your priorities and listen carefully to what your doctor is telling you. For instance, it may seem important to you to have a short hospital stay, so that you will not be separated from your other children for too long. Your doctor may take the more conservative view that even if the birth and your recovery are routine, it is important for you to have an extended period of rest and recuperation under the complete care of the hospital staff. Once you and the doctor understand each other's point of view, you may agree to make a final decision after the baby is born. That way, if you still want to return home after four or five days, your doctor will be satisfied that your recovery is well under way and you are not overestimating your ability to cope at home.

If you are hoping to see major changes in your doctor's or your hospital's policies, then it is essential that you start a dialogue with everyone concerned right now. (See Chapter Fifteen, "Support Groups: What Can You Do?" for a description of some ways to encourage these changes.) It will be essential for you to have intelligent, supportable reasons for the changes you are requesting. Merely saying that you would like it better that way is not effective unless the request is quite minor. If you approach your doctor at this first visit with a spirit of co-operation and open-mindedness, then your planning will be off to a good start.

## WHO SAYS I AM A HIGH RISK MOTHER?

If you are the inquisitive type, you may have discovered that you, like all women who are anticipating a Cesarean birth, are classified as "high risk." Many women worry that their doctor expects serious problems, or that there is something the doctor isn't telling them, when they see the words "high risk." However, the phrase does not mean what most women imagine. It is a label applied in every case where a routine vaginal delivery is not expected. The very fact that you will have a surgical delivery makes you "high risk" in medical parlance.

The use of the "high risk" label is mostly preventive. It reminds your doctor and anyone else who supports you during your pregnancy that your needs are not entirely the same as other mothers'. It may alert your doctor to the importance of helping you to prepare emotionally for this birth. It may cause him or her to exercise special care in making sure you do not become anemic, since this would create unnecessary additional burdens during surgery and your recovery period. By calling your pregnancy "high risk," the doctor may be helping himself or herself to avert some of the very risks that cause concern.

Occasionally, a mother who is high risk has known problems such as diabetes or hypertension that do create a significantly higher risk for her or her baby. If this is the case for you, your doctor will certainly be frank with you, and he or she will enlist your co-operation in taking every step possible to lessen these risks. Be sure to ask for a full discussion of any actual risks that your doctor is concerned about.

## THINKING WAY AHEAD

When this child is born, will your family be complete? If you think you may not want any more children, then you will want to consider having a tubal ligation ("having your tubes tied") at the same time that your Cesarean delivery is performed. There are distinct advantages to this, since it saves you the inconvenience of a separate procedure. There is also some slight statistical benefit, since you will be exposed to the risks associated with anesthesia only once. On the other hand, many couples who feel quite sure they want no more children still choose to delay sterilization. They may want to be sure that the baby is healthy, or they may want to have some experience with a family of this size before making a final decision. It is helpful to begin discussing this now, even though the birth is so far away, since it is a permanent measure.

## HELPING YOURSELF GET READY

Good nutrition, like motherhood itself, is something almost no one is against. Undoubtedly, you have every intention of taking good care of yourself during this pregnancy. You know that this is especially important for you as a Cesarean parent, because it will help to speed your recovery from surgery.

Yet, like all good intentions, it is easier said than done. You feel so tired during the early part of your pregnancy, and it isn't like the first time, when you could just take a nap. Now your older child has his own schedule and his own needs. By the time you think about what is for dinner, it is tempting to prepare whatever is easiest rather than whatever is healthiest.

This may be the time to learn how to use your slow cooker, so that the major share of food preparation can be done in the morning, when you are most energetic. And your husband can assume more of the responsibility. If he is already a gourmet cook, take advantage! If not, he can certainly prepare salads every night while you do the rest. And your two-year-old might love to "set the table," even if only a few spoons and forks at a time.

On the nights when you really need a break, pick one of the fast-food places that includes a salad bar and a choice of chicken or fish, then add milk and skip dessert. (If you think of this as a way of being good to yourself and an investment in your quick recovery from surgery, then you won't feel so deprived if you skip dessert.)

Exercise is another one of those activities that everyone greets with good intentions. Yet the mother of young children, though she may be on the go and feel tired much of the time, does not get enough of the right kinds of exercise unless she makes a special effort. If you're farsighted enough to be involved already in an activity like tennis or swimming, then you only need to keep on doing it for as long as your doctor will permit. But most of us are sadly out of shape, and pregnancy is not the time to launch a major offensive against your sagging form. Moderate, regular exercise will help you feel better during your pregnancy. And, like good nutrition, it is an investment in yourself and your quick recovery from surgery. There are some excellent books on exercise during pregnancy available now. (Please see bibliography.)

I have always struggled with my weight, and my first pregnancy was no exception. I gained thirty pounds, which I thought was pretty good. But it didn't come off as fast as I thought it would after the baby was born. In fact, ten of the extra pounds were still there two years later, when I got pregnant again. I knew it was too late to go on a diet, and I was kicking myself for not doing it when I could have.

This is also a good time to familiarize yourself with the exercises prescribed for Cesarean mothers after the baby is born. Some of these should be started as soon as your anesthetic has worn off, but you can't be expected to do them as effectively unless you and your husband have practiced before the birth.

## GETTING YOURSELF READY EMOTIONALLY

Since you already have had one Cesarean, you may expect yourself to feel like an "old pro" this time. Friends comment on how lucky you are to know exactly when the baby will arrive, so you can have everything ready. Yet there may be plenty of times when you don't feel lucky, or ready either. Looking back at your first pregnancy, maybe your surprise Cesarean wasn't bad after all. In some ways, ignorance was bliss.

There are many reasons why a second pregnancy carries more worries with it than the first one did. Some of them are common to everyone, no matter how the second baby will arrive. For instance, during your first pregnancy, you probably had a sense of wonder and elation at the miracle of life growing inside you. Although the pregnancy had its difficult moments, that sense of wonder probably carried you through the rough spots without much trouble. This time, though, some of the wonder is gone, so there is less to compensate for the trying times.

> The first time I got pregnant, I didn't really believe there was a baby in there. Of course I knew there was, I felt him move all the time, but some part of me thought it was all a dream. When he was finally born, I kept saying, "I can't believe it, I just can't believe it." Then when Sarah was born, I felt relieved but not so surprised. There was almost a letdown feeling, like I knew all along there would be a baby coming out, but I wished it didn't have to hurt so much.

Another factor that may be causing some difficulties with your second pregnancy is simply that it is your second pregnancy. Each baby's nine months in your uterus is a major physical event that takes its toll on you. It stands to reason that pregnancy will feel a little more wearing each time.

No doubt your older child is contributing his own complications to the picture. When you got pregnant the first time, you could just take a nap or eat out if you felt tired. But this time is quite different. Your budget or your toddler's refusal to sit in a high chair for longer than three minutes may prevent you from eating out. And more than one mother has discovered that her first child decided to stop taking naps just when the second one was on the way. It becomes more and more difficult to take good care of yourself and continue to do a good job in your other roles —mother, wife, housekeeper, employee, etc. If you are already concerned about how you will handle two children, it comes as an unpleasant shock to find that it isn't easy to handle one child and one pregnancy.

Cesarean parents have an additional source of anxiety that other parents do not, and that is the memory of the pain that was inevitably associated with the surgery last time. Research suggests that people who have already experienced a certain kind of pain may be more anxious, when they face that pain again, than people who are experiencing it for the first time. Although this may not be a major concern for you, it can be an underlying source of worry, which makes it a little harder to deal with all of the other normal anxieties connected with second pregnancies.

Sometimes a second Cesarean does not hurt as much as the first. This is apparently due to the fact that some of the nerves that were cut the first time do not completely return to their former level of functioning. On the other hand, some women report experiencing even more pain during subsequent Cesareans. There are two possible reasons for this: The first is that the postpartum uterine contractions (also called afterpains) are thought to cause more pain after subsequent pregnancies than they do after the first. The second is that some women do not feel as great an emotional "high" with subsequent deliveries, so the pain is more intrusive.

If you do have the possibility of a vaginal birth available to you, then uncertainty clouds all of your thoughts and plans. To be sure, a labor that results in vaginal delivery would be the best possible antidote to any negative feelings you had about your first birth experience. Yet your doctor is undoubtedly cautious about the prospects, and you almost don't dare to hope for a vaginal birth and then be disappointed yet another time. So you work hard at staying loose and adapting to whatever awaits you. As time goes on, you may feel that having the mode of delivery settled once and for all, even if it had to be another Cesarean, would be preferable to all this uncertainty.

With all of this, it should not be surprising if you find yourself coping with a host of worries. Often these are expressed in your asking a great many questions about what will happen to you and your baby.

> My girlfriend had a Cesarean too, but she hated just about every part of it. Compared to her, mine was great. I never felt cheated, because the baby was everything I dreamed of, and I knew he might not have made it if he came the usual way. But when I found out I was pregnant again, I got the jitters. I started worrying about every little thing that could go wrong. I had so many questions, and my doctor's appointments seemed so far apart at first.

Couples who are facing a repeat Cesarean often have more worries about the baby than they did the first time. This is common for second pregnancies, but may be more apparent with Cesarean families. The most likely explanation is that most couples had little time to anticipate their first Cesarean. Even with preparation, they have to absorb the fact that everything did not go in the routine fashion. It is quite natural, then, to worry about what new surprises might be waiting with this pregnancy.

If you actually have some condition that you know may affect the baby, then of course you will feel some continuing anxiety until the moment of birth. Your nine months of pregnancy may seem like ninety. Your worry is certainly unavoidable, although there are some steps you can take to ease your way through this time. One of the best is to reach out to family and friends for support. There will be many times when you are feeling optimistic and brave, and many times when you are too busy with the day-to-day business of living even to remember to worry. But at the times when you do feel scared, think about who you would like to talk to or share a cup of coffee with, and call her! Of course, it is also essential for you to share your concerns with your husband. However, most couples have one member who is a "worrier" and one who is a "reassurer," so you may find yourself having the same conversation many times: "I'm worried." "Don't worry, everything will be fine." "But I'm worried." "Don't worry . . . ," etc.

Whether your worries are the vague fears every parent feels or the specific concerns of parents facing medical complications, you may find it difficult to latch onto a sympathetic, understanding supporter. Your partner, your doctor, and your friends may not understand your mixed feelings, or they may feel helpless to reassure you. Both your husband and your doctor share your wish that this baby could be born without any risk and without your experiencing any pain. So, when you express your fears, they are uncomfortably reminded of something they wish were not true, yet cannot change. This is a good time to find other Cesarean mothers to talk to, since many of them have had the same normal feelings that you are having now. And if you live in a large urban area, there are probably childbirth preparation classes specifically for Cesarean couples available at the hospital or through your childbirth education group.

> I couldn't see the point of classes. We already had one Cesarean, so why go to classes? But the more pregnant I got, the more questions we had. So we decided to sign up after all.

You probably will continue to have anxious moments until the baby is born. In addition to latching onto some sympathetic listeners, you can help yourself by becoming as informed as possible and planning as much of the birth as your circumstances allow. Though you can't make the baby come any sooner, you can have an important role in determining the details of his arrival.

# PREPARING YOUR CHILDREN

A new brother or sister will enrich your child's life as well as yours. But every parent worries about the best way to prepare their older child for the baby's arrival.

Much depends on your child's age. Preschoolers have very little concept of time, and so it is important not to emphasize the baby's birth too soon. Your pregnancy should not be a secret, since children usually sense that something is going on, but the real excitement should be reserved for much later.

If you are planning to make major changes in your older child's life, it is best to begin as soon as possible. Toilet training is more likely to last through the baby's arrival if it is well established before the birth. If this seems too soon, then wait until the baby has come and a new family equilibrium has been achieved before you even attempt training. If your older child will be giving up his crib to the baby, make the change early in your pregnancy and store the crib for a while before putting it in the baby's room.

Once the baby arrives, you probably will be restricted from heavy lifting. That restriction includes not lifting toddlers! In preparation for this time, it is a good idea to teach your older child how to climb in and out of his crib, if he will still use it, and his high chair. This is easiest if you place another chair next to the crib or high chair, then encourage your older child to venture out. Some children are delighted, while others want to remain dependent on you a little longer. Other kinds of independence such as dressing himself can be encouraged, but with the same risk that the older child will balk. Some of this newfound independence tends to be "forgotten" temporarily when the baby arrives, but it will come back.

Some children have a lot of questions about pregnancy, while others ask none. It helps to have a book for children that shows the baby's development at different stages of pregnancy. If your child does ask questions, keep your answers short and simple.

> First Carrie asked me how the baby got inside me. I knew she would, and I had thought about how to answer her, but hadn't come up with anything that satisfied me. It was too late then, so I just did the best I could. I said that I already had an egg inside me, and Daddy put a sperm in me, and the egg and sperm combined to make a baby. She seemed satisfied, and I was relieved to have the ice broken.

It is important to be honest with your child, even in areas that make you feel uncomfortable. Some Cesarean parents have a particularly difficult time explaining to their older child how the baby comes out. They worry that the idea of Mommy being cut will frighten the child. It seems best to tell your children, "Most babies come out through an opening in their mother's body called the vagina. But some babies, like you and like our new baby, come out through a different opening that the doctor makes. When the baby is big enough to be born I will go to the hospital and the doctor will make an opening and take the baby out." Some children want to know if this hurts. Again, honesty tempered by reassurance is the best approach. "The doctor gives me special medicine so that it doesn't hurt when he makes the opening and takes the baby out. Later on, it hurts for a while. When I come home with the baby it will still be sore. But they give me more medicine to help me feel better. And it is a very small hurt compared to how happy we are to have you!"

Once children understand that you will be leaving home in order to have the new baby, they become concerned about the separation and who will care for them while you are gone. If a grandparent or baby sitter who is familiar to your child will be there, then your child will feel reassured. If your helper is relatively unknown, it is wise to ask her to come to the house several times in the days right before you leave, so that she and your older child can become acquainted. Grandparents who live some distance from you and haven't visited for several months should be considered part of the "unfamiliar" category, and it would be ideal for them to arrive early.

It is also helpful to prepare your older child for what the baby will look like and act like when he first comes home. Children need to know that little babies only eat, sleep, cry, and need to have their diapers changed. If you will be breast-feeding, explain briefly what this will look like too. It is helpful to be frank about the fact that babies require a lot of attention and are not a lot of fun to play with at first. In addition, you may want to give your older child a role in caring for the baby, such as bringing you a clean diaper, and describe how much it means to you to have an older child who can help out. The more your older child feels included, the less strain there will be.

When it is almost time to go to the hospital, you should begin preparing your older child for the specific details of what his experience will be. If he can visit, describe what that may be like, including the fact that he may feel sad when he has to leave. If he cannot visit, it may help to keep a calendar and mark off each day until your return. Some mothers have found it helpful to make tape recordings for the older child to listen to while they are gone. Children under three may be confused and distressed when they hear your voice but cannot find you. But older children may get a great deal of enjoyment from hearing you read their favorite stories or sing songs on the tapes. Rather than have them be a surprise, it is better to make the tapes with the child present, and then play them several times before you go to the hospital, so he can begin to understand that it works like his favorite records.

Some Cesarean mothers worry about the moment when they see their older child for the first time after the baby's birth. They fear that the child may want to rush toward them and climb onto their lap right away. This is a good time to prepare your child for the fact that you will feel sore and can only cuddle very carefully. You can even rehearse your first meeting, showing the child how you will place a pillow on your lap and carefully help him climb up.

## WHERE OH WHERE DID MY SEX LIFE GO?

Sexual intimacy, like pregnancy and parenthood, is an intensely personal experience. Although we all make adjustments in our sexual behavior to deal with other factors in our lives, what is helpful to some may not be to others. During your first pregnancy, you undoubtedly experienced important changes in your sex life. Even if your desire for sex was not affected by the pregnancy, you probably found it necessary to be creative and find new ways to achieve sexual satisfaction. Once the baby was born and you felt comfortable enough to resume sexual relations, you had new adjustments to make—how to cope with the endless distractions that a new baby creates. For some, this becomes a problem only as the baby gets older and sleeps less. Other parents find just the fact that the baby is in the next room has some impact on their feelings about themselves and their sexuality.

Now, with your next pregnancy, you will be going through another period of adjustment. Like the last, some creativity and imagination are helpful. Unlike the last, however, you may be aware of many more feelings that detract from your sex life. You are more tired, more worried about the actual delivery, more aware of your body, and concerned that once again you will have a big incision and some soreness to reckon with. Some people find that they feel particularly shaky and vulnerable after surgery. They want to protect their body, keep it covered and secure. The touches that once might have been soothing now feel like invasions. When you are expecting a repeat Cesarean, it is not uncommon for these feelings to occur before the surgery, both as a response to pregnancy itself and also in anticipation of the operation.

None of these feelings need be fatal to your sex life, as long as you understand that they are normal and allow yourself lots of time to achieve a new balance and equilibrium. If your sex life was terrific, it can be really scary to see it seem to fall apart. And there are some aspects of it that won't come back for a long time. Once you have more than one young child you are sentenced to have sex together in the bedroom with the door closed late at night or early in the morning. The prospect of getting the children all to nap at once seems dim. Long, romantic Sunday afternoons can be recaptured only at the price of a hotel room. If your sex life wasn't terrific to begin with, you may feel that your last hope of improving it is disappearing as this baby's day of birth comes nearer.

Jack kept saying that it would be OK to try some new positions. He didn't seem to understand that I felt bigger than a whale. No matter what position we used, it meant I had to get down on the bed and then get up again afterward, and that alone seemed like a major project. But I got scared about how bad he would feel if I said no again. I felt like I had been pregnant forever.

There is no getting past the fact that this is a stressful time, and some parts of your relationship may temporarily suffer. It may be helpful to concentrate on the long-range view. You will not be pregnant forever, and the experiences you will share in these next months will add to your family's foundation. There will be a turning point—perhaps when the baby first starts sleeping through the night, or when spring comes and you can get outdoors with the children, or maybe as soon as your six-week postpartum checkup. Whenever it comes, it will mark the time when you know this is really worth all the work and worry.

Jay insisted that we should have some time alone together. I was weaning Kim, so I knew we would be able to get away, but part of me dreaded it. I knew that "time alone together" meant sex, and I sure didn't feel sexy. So we got to the motel, and I said I wanted to eat first. He had three cocktails and I had two. When we got back to the room, we watched TV and dozed off without ever making love. But the next morning was a different story. With all that time and no interruptions, it was just wonderful. Better than our honeymoon, because we knew what we were doing. And when we got back home the next day, the kids were happy as clams. And they looked so good to me, I was ready for motherhood again.

## AS THE DAY APPROACHES

In the final part of your pregnancy, a different kind of planning becomes important. By now, you and your husband and your doctor have achieved some basic understandings about what the main features of this birth will be. You know, to the extent that you can know, when the baby will be born (or what further steps will be necessary to determine the birth date), what kind of anesthesia is planned, whether your husband can be present in the delivery room or afterward in the recovery room, etc. Now you will want to focus on some details that will assure you that everything is ready.

Give some thought now to the roles your helper and your husband will play. Does the person who will be doing laundry know how to use your washing machine? If your helper will be cooking, are there things she should know about the family's tastes? Is it more important for your husband to be with you in the hospital during the evening hours, or for him to be home for the older child's bedtime?

> For the first baby, I took time off from work and spent most of it in the hospital with Debbie and the baby. I felt good that I could be there, especially when she couldn't get around very much. I even enjoyed going back to the quiet apartment at night after I left the hospital. But when the second one came I just felt exhausted and not very useful. Jason was giving my mother-in-law a hard time about going to bed at night, and I didn't know what to tell her about how to handle it. Debbie was pretty laid up and couldn't really keep the new baby in the room with her unless I was there to help. I couldn't be two places at once. And on top of it all, they called with some questions from work and I got the feeling they didn't really like me being out for the whole two weeks during the busy season.

The ideal way to prepare your helper is to spend some time with her before you go to the hospital. That way, she can cement her relationship with your older child, and you can give her a clear picture of what you expect her to do. Lists are essential! Your helper will profit from a written description of the daily routines, so that she can maintain things in their usual fashion as much as possible. She will need a list of neighbors, your child's pediatrician, emergency numbers, etc. Your husband may not need quite so many details, but he, too, may need to be reminded of daily routines. If you are really organized, you may have menus planned and meals frozen in advance. If so, there needs to be a list for these too.

Probably the best preparation for you at this point is to dust off your flexibility and sense of humor. No matter how much you plan, things will happen in your absence. Your son will be sent to nursery school in the one shirt you didn't manage to mend before the baby came. Your husband will ignore the meatloaf you carefully made and froze, and bring home lots of pizzas instead. Your mother-in-law will decide to surprise you by rearranging the living room furniture.

## WHAT IF LABOR STARTS?

Sometimes women who are awaiting a planned Cesarean go into labor. Since your childbirth preparation classes were long ago, you may have forgotten the signs. Aside from contractions, which usually can be identified, you may have a discharge as your mucus plug (sometimes tinged with blood) is passed. Or, if your membranes rupture spontaneously, you may feel a steady dribble or even a sudden rush of fluid. Some women experience a backache at the beginning of labor. The important thing is not to wait, but to call your doctor if you think there is the smallest possibility that you are starting labor.

It is a good idea to have a plan for what to do if labor starts. If you and your doctor have agreed to use the start of labor as a way of knowing when the baby is ready for delivery, then such a plan is essential. Who will care for your older child? How will you get to the hospital? Do you know how to contact your husband throughout the day? If he may be unavailable, who will be the backup person to support you until he can arrive?

If labor does begin, you should not eat or drink anything, since surgery is probably in your near future.

## EMOTIONS JUST BEFORE BIRTH DAY

Let's get this over with! You probably remember feeling this way the last time too. But that time there was some fun associated with the suspense of wondering when the baby would appear. Now you know that you have six weeks more to wait, and that seems endless. Once you may have wanted a boy or a girl more than anything. Now the sex of the baby does not seem to matter as much as having a healthy baby of either sex.

Although you keep busy with the care of your older child and the last stages of planning and preparation, some seemingly strange fears may surface at this time. Will the baby be all right? Will I be all right? What if I die? What if something terrible happens at home while I am away? Although we do not entirely understand why women have these fears, we do know that they are entirely normal. Perhaps the emotional upheaval they represent is the first stage of the family reorganizing to welcome its new member. In any case, although these fears may be persistent, they almost never come true. Instead, they simply go away as the birth finally occurs and you turn to the practical demands of your new situation.

Welcome, baby, at last!

## FOURTEEN

# Father-Attended Cesarean Birth

## WHO LET HIM IN HERE?

The practice of allowing fathers to attend vaginal deliveries began almost by accident. When the childbirth preparation movement got its start in North America, its purpose was simply to teach women techniques that would improve their birth experience and lessen their need for medication. The childbirth instructor was usually also the labor coach for her students. As time went on, the sheer numbers of women who flocked to childbirth instructors made it impossible for the instructor always to act as coach, and so husbands were recruited to attend classes and learn the coach's role.

These days, the opportunity to share the baby's birth is an essential part of childbirth preparation for most couples.

I asked Tom if he wanted to come with me to the classes. I had my fingers crossed that he would say yes. He said he honestly didn't know if he could go through the whole thing with me, but he was willing to go to the classes and try it. Seeing the movie convinced both of us that being together was the only way to go.

## BUT THIS IS MAJOR SURGERY

When a Cesarean delivery is necessary and the father is asked to wait outside, couples who had planned to be together are almost universally disappointed. For some, the separation is the most difficult part of the entire experience.

The wish of Cesarean couples to be together for their baby's birth is one of the most common, yet controversial and misunderstood aspects of Cesarean birth. So many reasons are given by doctors and hospitals who oppose father-attended Cesareans that it is difficult even to list them all. Among the more common are: What if the father faints? What if he gets upset at seeing his wife operated on and starts to interfere? What if something goes wrong before his very eyes? What if the father misunderstands something that happens and decides to sue the doctor?

On the more practical side, some doctors argue that the room in which Cesareans are done is too small to accommodate another person. Some say that two more persons would be required: the father, and an extra nurse to help out if he fainted or had a problem. Infection is a concern, and it may be argued that each new person is a potential source of bacteria. Anesthesiologists, who work near the mother's head where the father would be seated, worry that the father might interfere with their work or take up needed space.

Finally, some doctors simply say that having the father present would make them nervous, and they prefer not to add anyone to the scene who might distract them or interfere by producing additional tension.

Occasionally, Cesarean couples are viewed as morbid or weird if they ask to be together for the baby's birth. The father who is willing to be present when his wife is being operated on is thought to be asking for something almost indecent. Although these ideas are seldom verbalized to the couple's face, they may be spoken behind their back as opponents of father-attended birth search for ways to justify their opposition.

Finally, couples who wish to be together may find that they are being told no, but it is almost impossible to find out who is against the idea, what the reasons are, and where the final authority lies. You may hear, "I am not opposed to this, but ——— will never agree to it." Obstetricians say this about anesthesiologists, nurses about hospital administrators, and so on. Since many professionals now set practice standards as a group, you may be told that your own doctor would like to allow you to be together, but it is impossible to get all the other doctors who have obstetrical privileges at that hospital to go along. One of the most difficult of all situations to respond to is when almost everyone concerned is opposed to allowing the father to attend the birth, but each person has a different reason.

> It seemed like a simple enough request to me. We had been to-
> gether for the last one, and it never occurred to us that the hospital
> in our new area wouldn't allow it. Since it was just routine at the
> old place, I didn't really have to give it any thought. Now, with just
> about everyone sounding so negative or surprised that we wanted to
> be together, it took a lot of work just to organize our thoughts
> about why. It was obvious that a simple "Well, why not?" was not
> going to convince anyone. I really think if we hadn't already done
> it, we might have decided it was a silly idea and just given up. But I
> knew what it meant to both of us, so we kept meeting with people
> and talking and plugging along patiently.

## WHY COUPLES WANT TO BE TOGETHER

The situation facing Cesarean couples who wish to be together is virtually identical to the situation couples who wished to be together for their vaginal birth once faced. The same reasons are being given for keeping fathers in the waiting room. And the reasons are gradually being proven wrong in the same way that they were for vaginal births.

> I wasn't even scared. The first time I had a Cesarean I was convinced I was going to die, but for Becky I wasn't even scared. Jim held my hand the whole time and talked to me about how wonderful I was and what a beautiful baby we were going to have. I asked if they had started and the doctor said they almost had the baby already. When they lifted her out I gave a yell, feeling the pressure and then seeing her right there. We both were crying as they cleaned her up, and then they brought her for Jim to hold while I touched her face and counted all her fingers and toes. It was the most wonderful thing that has ever happened to us.

Most couples who wish to share their Cesarean birth, like those who wish to share vaginal birth, place a strong value on mutual support and sharing in all aspects of their relationship. For some, being together seems like a natural extension of everything they believed in when they decided to have a baby.

> My father didn't have much to do with us when we were kids. Really, he couldn't because he had to work two jobs to keep us going. But when I started thinking about being a father myself, I didn't want it to be that way. I went to the childbirth classes because I wanted this baby to know its father from the minute it got here.

For others, the most important aspect of a shared Cesarean is the support that the father can give the mother during the surgery. No matter how prepared the mother is, everyone feels some nervousness when a surgical birth is necessary. But the presence of the father can be the single element that makes the difference between the mother feeling confident or anxious at the time of birth. The issue of how the mother feels during the birth is not simply a matter of luxury. Extreme anxiety can actually interfere with the procedure.

If you are one of the very large number of couples who wish to share your Cesarean birth experience, you will be encouraged to know that the list of hospitals that offer this option is growing every day. There are many reasons why it is becoming more common, not the least of which is the pressure on hospitals from consumers. But pressure alone does not change the way medicine is practiced. The essential elements that have convinced doctors and hospitals to change their policies are that father-attended Cesarean births have important benefits, and they do not carry the risks that their opponents fear.

## THE EVIDENCE

In a recent study, doctors evaluated sixty-six Cesarean births that were attended by the father.[1] These were compared with a like number of births where the father did not attend. The two groups were chosen randomly, and matched to be sure that there were not any significant differences in the two populations. Fathers did not know until the last minute whether they would attend the birth. Both unexpected and planned Cesareans were included in the sample, and both repeat and first-time Cesareans were included. The fathers did not receive any formal preparation for the birth, except being told where to sit in the operating room.

Some of the most important results of the study are described by what did *not* happen during these births. No father became sick, fainted, or interfered in any way. Fathers did not obstruct the ability of the professionals attending the birth to complete their assigned tasks. In fact, although some staff members had been worried about the effects of the father's presence, the experiment was concluded earlier than was originally planned because the staff found shared Cesarean birth to be so preferable to the old way that they asked for the study to be stopped so that *all* fathers could begin attending the births!

The fathers' presence also did not affect the rate of complications connected with the birth. There were no postpartum infections in the group where fathers were present, and there was one

[1] G. Nolan, M. Gainer, P. Van Bonn. Unpublished data obtained through personal communication. This is a collaborative study done by the School of Nursing and the Obstetric Department at the University of Michigan, Ann Arbor.

infection among the mothers whose husbands were not present for the birth.

It is also interesting to note that the mothers whose husbands were present for the birth took slightly less medication for pain during the early recovery period than did the mothers whose husbands were not present. However, this difference was not great enough to be statistically significant.

Probably the most important finding of the study on father-attended births was this: Mothers whose partners were present at the birth reported significantly greater feelings of satisfaction with the birth itself and with their own recovery from the birth. Although further research is needed in this area, it seems likely that a mother's feelings about the baby's birth and her own recovery will become essential parts of her overall feelings about herself as a parent.

## WHAT IF SOMETHING GOES WRONG?

For anesthesiologists, the usual concern about fathers' presence is what would happen in the unlikely event that the mother has heart failure as a result of anesthesia. For the obstetrician and pediatrician, the worry is that the baby will have some problem at birth. There can be no denying that these problems do occur, if only extremely rarely.

> I heard the baby cry, and it sounded kind of funny to me. They had the equipment where I could watch, and I could hear them suctioning him. Jack asked how soon before he could hold the baby, and the pediatrician started saying that there was a problem with his breathing. Jack grabbed my hand and we both just watched and listened. It seemed like forever. I completely lost track of the fact that they were still working on me. Finally, they brought the baby over for a quick look. He looked a little blue, but I could see him moving and he seemed lively. The pediatrician said that he would go to the special nursery for treatment, and that the next few days would be the critical time. We decided that Jack would go to the nursery

while they finished with me. He came back as soon as I was in the recovery room and told me how the baby looked and what was happening. He even brought a little Polaroid picture of him in the incubator.

The question of what will happen in the event something goes wrong is more a question of values and philosophy than it is of right or wrong. The doctor who emphasizes the family aspect of birth and who expects parents to take a great deal of responsibility for their birth experience will welcome both their presences when a problem arises. In fact, from the start of the doctor's relationship with them, he or she will be concerned not only for the pregnant woman but for the entire family. The doctor will recognize that they prefer to function as a partnership whenever possible, and that they can support each other emotionally in a crisis, while necessary medical tasks are performed. He or she will have confidence in their ability to support each other in difficult times as well as in times of joy.

Other professionals place a high value on their right to deal with medical crises with the least possible amount of distraction. They feel that if the father is present when a crisis occurs, then the father's need for information and reassurance may detract from the immediate needs of the mother or baby for emergency care. Sometimes medical professionals feel most comfortable when they can communicate a sense of certainty and of being in control to their patients. A crisis, filled with unpredictability, makes it more difficult for the professional to behave in this reassuring way.

If your doctor is willing to consider allowing you to be together for your baby's birth, he or she may wish to plan for every possibility with you, including the slim chance that something may go wrong. Although the topic is not a comfortable one, your doctor's concern on this score is understandable. Some doctors are more willing to let fathers be present if the couple is willing to sign a written agreement reviewing all the contingencies and stating that the husband will leave the Cesarean delivery room without delay if he is asked to do so.

## WHAT ABOUT MALPRACTICE PROBLEMS?

The rumors about Cesarean births and malpractice suits are wide-spread. When couples express a wish to be together for a Cesarean, "legal issues" are often mentioned as one reason why the father should not be present. There is the implication that someone might sue someone, although exactly who would be sued or why is left somewhat unclear. Occasionally, couples may be told that the father's presence is not legal. (There is a law in one area prohibiting anyone but medical personnel from being present during surgery. It was created to keep medical-equipment sales-men out of the operating room. That state's Supreme Court re-fused to hear the case of one Cesarean father who challenged the law because it excluded him.)

The same issues were raised when couples first asked to share a vaginal delivery. Based on that trend, there are some clear legal issues that can be pinpointed. There is no evidence that the fa-ther's presence affects the question of whether a suit will be filed by the parents if something goes wrong. What is true is simply that a father who has attended the birth will probably testify in court if a suit is filed. The father is likely to be an impassioned but medically uninformed witness who, it is argued, might sway the jury in the family's favor.

The same circumstances apply to Cesarean birth, and since the trend is to allow fathers to attend Cesareans, there undoubtedly will soon be a suit by parents against a doctor where the birth was surgical and the father witnessed the delivery. However, it seems unlikely that the father's presence will serve to increase the number of suits filed. Some have argued that the father who is present for a Cesarean birth where something goes wrong is less likely to sue, since he can observe the medical team in action firsthand and appreciate their efforts in an emergency. However, the father's presence will make those few suits that are filed more complicated because the father will offer testimony as a witness.

The malpractice crisis in North America hurts health care providers and consumers alike. It creates an atmosphere of conservatism and distrust. Few couples would ever sue their doctor, and few doctors are guilty of malpractice, yet all are affected by the problem. Fortunately, fathers now routinely attend vaginal births in most areas, despite the legal concerns that once accompanied this practice. The same trend has been set in motion for Cesarean families.

## WHAT ABOUT GENERAL ANESTHESIA?

Even hospitals where fathers are encouraged to attend most Cesarean births typically bar the father when general anesthesia is used. The reason is simple: He cannot perform his major role, support of the mother, when she is unconscious throughout the procedure. Although this seems sensible at first glance, there are good reasons to include the father when the mother will not be awake. One of the best is that the father's attachment to the baby, which apparently develops in much the way that the mother's does, can begin sooner and perhaps be enhanced when he is allowed to be present and hold the baby immediately.

> Even though I had to stay on that stool and out of the way, I was able to see most of what was happening. Then the doctor handed her to me. The nurse asked me her name, and I said it was Adrienne, and the name seemed just right to me. She was just beautiful, just like an Adrienne should be.

In addition to the direct benefits to the father, his presence may have some advantages for the mother as well. There are anecdotal reports that show that some Cesarean mothers who have a general anesthetic have more difficulties with their postpartum adjustment than mothers who are awake during the birth. This problem is probably most characteristic of women who, during their pregnancy, placed a strong value on their own participation in and mastery of the birth. When they are not even "there" while the baby is being delivered, they are forced to fill in the gaps themselves, imagining the baby's arrival and their own role in it. If their husband has been present as the family's representative, then the emotional missing link between pregnancy and baby is more easily resolved.

> They wheeled me into the room and got everything set up. Doug came in, looking a little strange behind that mask, but I knew that he was grinning the way he does when he's excited. He held my hand until I fell asleep. Then I don't remember anything until I started to come out of it, and there he was again. No mask this time, just the grin. He said, "It's a girl, we got our girl!" It took me a minute to really absorb what he said, but then I think I started grinning too. When I got back to my room and they brought her in, he said, "Cynthia Ann, meet your mother. Mom, this is your new daughter, Cynthia Ann." I got to laughing until my stitches hurt. I never had the little doubts I had with our first one about whether this was the right baby.

## WHAT ABOUT AN UNEXPECTED CESAREAN?

Many hospitals that allow fathers to be present for some Cesarean births maintain a policy that the Cesarean must be planned (some exclude all but repeat Cesareans) so that the father can be prepared for what he will hear and see. Often the same facilities make special Cesarean birth preparation classes available, so that a father may become prepared for a Cesarean birth in the same ways that fathers are now preparing for vaginal births.

The value of preparation cannot be underestimated. However, although the father may feel more comfortable when he knows what to expect, there is no evidence that an unprepared father is any more likely to become upset or interfere than one who understands everything that is happening. Increasingly, traditional childbirth preparation classes are including extensive materials on both modes of birth, so that a father knows what to expect in a

Cesarean birth. Until this sort of preparation is widespread, there will be some surprised and uncomfortable fathers. However, their own reports indicate that most fathers prefer to be present, even though unprepared, rather than excluded from the birth.


## THE VALUE OF SHARED BIRTH

Although the scientific data are not available yet, the firsthand experiences of thousands of parents are convincing evidence that father-attended Cesarean births help to form the foundation for a healthy family. Parents who greet their Cesarean baby together feel more satisfied, and their contentment must surely contribute to their ability to grow through the milestone of childbirth.

Expectant parents want a healthy baby more than anything else. But most parents also want an emotionally gratifying beginning as a family. Supporters of shared Cesarean birth believe that it is not necessary to choose between the two.

# FIFTEEN

# Support Groups: What Can You Do?

## STARTING A GROUP

Once you have a detailed understanding of Cesarean birth, you may feel satisfied enough to go on to parenthood without any further attention to the way the baby arrived. For many parents, simply becoming informed is the key to a happy, rewarding Cesarean. But some parents choose to become involved in a Cesarean parents' support group, both because they want further support for themselves and because they want to encourage changes in the ways in which Cesareans are typically handled in their area. In fact, there are about 150 such support groups in the United States that are independently organized, and probably hundreds more Cesarean support committees within the local childbirth education groups. If you are interested in such a group, start by finding out if one already exists in your area. Your physician, childbirth educator, or hospital maternity nurses probably will know what is available.

Most new parents want to tell their birth story over and over. For Cesarean parents, the opportunities to talk to someone who really understands may be limited, so they often are bursting to talk when they first attend a support group meeting. If the birth was particularly traumatic, they may need to repeat some parts of the story many times before they emotionally accept what happened to them. Others may come to the group anticipating a first Cesarean, and seeking information and reassurance from couples who already have had the experience. Often people who join support groups have a strong wish to change whichever aspect of the birth was least satisfying for them.

> Seth was three months old. We had it planned that I would get pregnant again in about two years. I figured that was two years to work toward getting the hospital to allow my husband to be with me for the birth. With other hospitals in nearby towns starting to do it, it seemed like our chances were pretty good.

If there is not a group in your area, perhaps you can be the catalyst for starting one. If you do, you will experience all the frustrations that are common to volunteer organizations, plus a few more, because your group will almost certainly tread on some toes in your community. But the personal and social rewards are tremendous.

> When I first went to the group, all I knew was that Luke's birth didn't happen the way we wanted. As I listened to other women's stories, the knot in my stomach went away. I felt such relief to know that others were disappointed and upset too. It gave me some perspective and I began to genuinely appreciate the parts of it that were good.

## WHAT GROUPS CAN DO

Some groups limit themselves to the kinds of personal and practical support that individual Cesarean families need. Many also organize projects that will benefit everyone who has a Cesarean, regardless of whether they join the group or not. Ideally, the ultimate goal of every group should be to make Cesarean birth such a prepared, joyous experience that a group is not needed. Realistically, though, Cesarean birth is largely subject to the same ignorance and fears that were associated with vaginal birth twenty years ago. Small wonder the Cesarean support movement is growing so rapidly. Groups that manage to stay organized and intent on their goals are having a tremendous impact on the way Cesareans are done in the United States.

The most successful support groups chose one or two, or at most three projects to work on at one time. Usually the projects are simply those that capture the interest of most members. For those who don't want to organize a project, there are plenty of tasks remaining that are important, such as getting to know new members, and perhaps arranging coffees so that three or four new members can have an opportunity to tell each other what happened to them.

The following chart lists most of the family centered alternatives that different Cesarean couples have enjoyed. Support groups often find it helpful to circulate a list such as this in order to stimulate discussion among members and to set priorities for group projects. Taken as a whole, the chart demonstrates that Cesarean birth can be family centered in many of the same ways that vaginal birth can be. Probably no hospital offers all these alternatives, and few couples would find them all appealing. Nor is the chart meant to imply that there is a right or a wrong way to have a Cesarean delivery. Rather, the chart will stimulate your thinking about what is possible, and help you establish your priorities.

I couldn't believe it. After the first baby was born, I felt left out when my friends would talk about their deliveries. After the Cesarean group started, we seemed to have our own unspoken contest to see who could have the "best" Cesarean. Everyone was so enthused about bonding and closeness. Well, I didn't want to nurse the baby right away, and I wasn't sure I wanted to even be awake for the birth. I finally spoke up about it at a meeting, and somebody else supported me. After that I felt better—about me and the group.

# FAMILY-CENTERED CESAREAN BIRTH

| ALTERNATIVE | COMMENTS |
|---|---|
| **Prior to birth** | |
| Traditional childbirth classes that fully cover Cesarean birth. | Increasingly, material on Cesarean birth is taught in parallel with that on vaginal birth, instead of being reserved for an isolated portion of one class. |
| Separate Cesarean childbirth preparation classes for couples who anticipate a Cesarean. | Best when co-led by an instructor and Cesarean parent, or an instructor who has had a Cesarean. |
| Hospital admission on the day of the birth, or admission the night before—but parents to be leave hospital and go out to dinner. | If couple arrives late, the entire surgery schedule for that day is disrupted. Promptness is a must! |
| Partial "prep"—shaving abdomen and top inch or two of pubic hair only. | Less unpleasant for mother; lessens itching and improves body image. |
| Full explanation of purpose and effects of preoperative medication, including sleeping pills, tranquilizers, etc. | This is the patient's right to "informed consent." |
| Choice of anesthesia between regional and general, unless medically inadvisable. | Some areas have anesthesiologists experienced in only one form of anesthesia. |

## At the Time of Birth

Birth and recovery room stay on maternity service rather than general surgical unit.

Transverse ("bikini") skin incision.

Father or supportive other person present for birth.

Mirror placed so that mother can see birth.

Drape lowered so that mother can see baby at birth.

Pictures taken of the birth.

Mother given verbal description of the birth as it occurs.

Baby suctioned and evaluated within mother's range of vision.

Mother has one arm free to touch baby as soon as possible.

If father is absent, he is notified as soon as baby is born.

## Immediately After Birth

Mother, father, and baby together in the recovery room; mother hold and nurse baby if desired.

---

In some hospitals, this would require knocking out some walls and installing new equipment.

Much more acceptable cosmetically.

See Chapter Fourteen, "Father-Attended Cesarean Birth."

Not everyone wants to see themselves operated on!

Some concerns about loss of protection of sterile operative area.

Flash cameras usually prohibited.

Helps mother to feel her importance. Avoids "shop talk" and keeps her included.

Visual reassurance to mother of baby's reality.

Tactile reassurance of baby's reality. Early contact promotes feelings of attachment.

Usually done by pediatrician or nurse en route to nursery with baby. Lessens anxiety for father.

Mother probably more comfortable now than when she returns to her room.

| ALTERNATIVE | COMMENTS |
|---|---|
| Baby placed in special care nursery only if required by his individual condition. | Conveys confidence to parents in baby's well-being. |
| Father or other helper present in mother's room whenever desired. | Identifies father as essential family member, not visitor. Promotes father's attachment to baby. |
| Modified rooming-in according to mother's needs and availability of helper. | Encourages mother to take responsibility for baby, at the same time permitting mother enough rest. |
| Baby's crib marked so that nurses recall that birth was a Cesarean each time baby is brought to mother's room. | Assures mother necessary help getting baby in and out of crib, changing positions, etc. |
| Bedside help from nurses in caring for baby. | Helps mother overcome feelings of helplessness. |
| Cesarean roommate if desired. | Although she will be more sympathetic, she may not be able to be as helpful to you as a roommate who delivered vaginally would. |
| Electrical bed. | Easier on mothers, nurses, and other helpers. |
| Wheelchair available to mother if baby in special care nursery. | Mother will imagine things much worse than what she will actually see if she is allowed to visit. |
| Support and education for breast-feeding mothers. | Good for all mothers, but some practical tips are especially helpful for Cesarean mothers. |

| | |
|---|---|
| Mother in room close to nursing station and nursery. | Easiest if the floor is not overcrowded. |
| Mother graduates to solid diet as soon as her individual condition permits. | Solid food does wonders for the morale! |

### Later Postpartum Period

| | |
|---|---|
| Sibling visitation. | Especially beneficial to families when mother's hospital stay is longer. |
| Nursing staff introduces Cesarean families to each other. | Helps you know you are not alone. |
| Nursing staff provides postpartum teaching about Cesareans, using visual aides. | Research shows that postpartum teaching improves mothers' satisfaction with birth and recovery. |
| Length of stay determined by individual needs. | Some mothers want to prolong the period of being cared for. Others can't wait to get home. |
| Literature about Cesarean birth available to take home. | Most couples have many questions between hospital stay and six-week checkup. Literature serves as a useful reference. |
| Family informed about posthospital services, including Cesarean support group and visiting nurses; phone numbers supplied. | Eases the transition to home. Acknowledges the normal need for ongoing postpartum support. |
| Full discussion of all aspects of their individual birth experience with both parents and doctor prior to hospital discharge. | Encourages parents to understand and accept the Cesarean and promotes realistic expectations for the early recovery period. |

## GETTING A GROUP STARTED

You may begin alone, or perhaps you already know one or two
people who would be willing to help you start a group. All it
takes to organize the first meeting is a lot of time and a small
amount of money for postage and refreshments. It helps to set the
date of the meeting far enough in advance to allow yourself time
for both telephone and written publicity. Doctors' offices should
be notified by a phone call to the nurse or receptionist, followed
by a card that can be posted in the office.

Childbirth instructors are another valuable link to interested
people, and they often have a newsletter that is sent to couples
who have recently taken classes. In addition, you should contact
local newspapers, and TV and radio stations that carry public
service announcements. Be sure that you give your name and
phone number to everyone you contact, in case they have any
questions. For these early contacts, it is appropriate to state the
purposes of the group very generally, such as "education and support for the Cesarean family." The membership will define what
specific kinds of support they are most concerned about.

Usually the only thing that can be accomplished at the first
meeting is to give everyone a chance to tell their story. This is essential, and if it takes all night, that's fine. The group exists for its
members first, so start right out listening and supporting each
other. There should be someone leading the meeting, but she
should intervene only if there is a danger that not everyone will
be heard. You may want to consider using nametags if you have a
large group. There should be a signup sheet circulating with a
simple statement at the top such as, "I am interested in knowing
about meetings of the Cesarean support group" with a place for
names, addresses, and phone numbers. Also, it isn't uncommon
for people at the first meeting to volunteer to help organize the
next one, but if they don't, ask!

During the first meeting, you may find it helpful to jot down the concerns of everyone there. This doesn't need to be elaborate; just a few phrases will do, such as "Wish I had been better prepared"; "Hospital was great, but I never expected to be so tired at home"; "Wish we could have been together," etc. If you have access to copying equipment, run off copies of this list of concerns and distribute it at the next meeting and to future new members.

## BUILDING MOMENTUM

The next few meetings of the group are important in several ways. This will be the time when the original members of the group are getting to know each other and establishing some trust and personal ties. At the same time, new members will keep appearing and will have their own needs. Many groups report that only about 60 per cent of the people who come to a meeting return for subsequent meetings. This can be discouraging if you don't expect it. It may mean that the group is not what they are looking for, but it may also mean that they got what they needed the first time and have no desire to return. As time goes on, a core of faithfuls will emerge.

One of the main things that makes a group succeed is its ability to strike a balance between the personal needs of members and the completion of projects that the group undertakes. Often group members find themselves needing to talk about themselves. If other members are too busy to listen, everyone may end up feeling unsatisfied. Yet both aspects of the group are vital. It may be useful to separate the two functions—personal support and completing tasks—in some way. Some groups are big enough to sponsor mothers' support groups and simultaneously to hold monthly business meetings devoted entirely to projects. Others have arranged their meetings so that new members come forty-five minutes early, and are greeted and invited to share their concerns with several old members who volunteer for this role. Then the business meeting begins and is open to all. Other groups try to push their way through the business agenda in the first hour, encouraging a more informal exchange at the end of each meeting.

No matter how your group copes with this question, it seems that both personal interchange and some projects are essential if the group is to provide the broad base of support that Cesarean families need. Although most groups avoid elaborate organizational structures, it is necessary to establish some committees and have responsibilities clearly assigned. Usually those who start groups absorb the initial expenses. Once the group is established, you may wish to collect a small amount of dues to pay for paper, postage, phone, and refreshments.

## CHOOSING PROJECTS

No matter what the group chooses for its projects, the first thing you will need is information. Usually the following outline can be applied to almost any issue the group chooses to examine:

1. What are the local practices, and why?
2. What alternatives are there, at least in theory?
3. What medical as well as personal reasons are there for seeking alternatives?
4. Who has the authority to change the local practices?

For instance, perhaps the group members discover that only general anesthesia is used for Cesareans in your area. There can be many reasons for this. It may be that no one is experienced enough with regional anesthesia. It may be that all the anesthesiologists practice as a group, and have chosen this as their standard of practice. Whatever the reasons, you need to understand each of them clearly. At the same time, someone should review the available literature on Cesarean birth and become a lay expert on the alternatives to general anesthesia. This much alone may take several months. Then, if your group or a committee of the group continues to place a high priority on making regional anesthesia available, you will have to begin a dialogue with those who have the authority to implement your preferences. Personal feelings carry little weight until medical issues are resolved, so you must be prepared to give evidence that what you are asking for is not just your whims. Sounds like a lot of work? It is! But it can be worthwhile.

## RELATIONSHIPS WITH THE PROFESSIONAL COMMUNITY

The most effective groups are those who have a medical adviser or perhaps even an entire advisory board. These should be sympathetic professionals chosen from the fields of obstetrics, pediatrics, anesthesiology, family medicine, or childbirth education. The main role of an adviser is to provide information, both about his or her specialty and about the complexities of the health care delivery system. No adviser can do your work for you, but he or she can do such things as suggest journal articles for you to read, or help you understand why things are done the way they are.

> During the question-and-answer period, we asked Dr. Williams why they shaved the whole pubic area, even though the incision was up in the abdomen. We thought if we explained how awful the itching was when the hair grew back, he could just pass the word and they could change it. Instead, he started talking about some committee at the hospital that had responsibility for maintaining sterile procedures, and said the committee probably had made a policy requiring total shaves. Incredible! We thought it would be so simple.

In addition to the information they provide, advisers have the distinct advantage of lending credibility to the group. It is important, though, that your advisers and you have the freedom and trust in each other to disagree. Advisers may not share all your goals or approve of all your tactics, and it is essential that you get their advance permission before publicly associating them with the group's projects.

Regardless of whether you are dealing with a sympathetic professional or one whose views are at the opposite end of the pole, courtesy and a willingness to listen are essential if you are to succeed. You may find yourself in adversary relationships with the powers that be. Most of us are uncomfortable in such a role, and so we may give up too soon or call in the cannons when verbal negotiations would do. You may be right, but that is little consolation if you have alienated the people whose willingness to listen is essential for your success.

## TACTICS

Once you have done your homework, then the first tactic for implementing change is simply to ask for it. Approach the person or persons in authority and ask for a discussion of your chosen issue. Present your point of view and listen carefully to what is said to you. Return to your group to report and plan further. Probably more meetings will be required with the various people involved. If the time stretches on and little is accomplished, a letter-writing campaign by your members may help. Letters should be short and to the point, explaining what changes you wish to see, and why. A sentence to the effect, "As consumers, this issue is so important that it will play a significant role in our choice of a maternity service for future births" will alert your listener to the possibility that you will use another facility in order to get the kind of birth experience you want. If there are members of the group who are willing to go outside the immediate community— for instance, so that the father can attend the birth—then this should be pointed out too.

In some communities, further pressure through the media can be effective. For instance, you might ask each member who writes a letter to the local hospital to send a copy of the letter to the newspaper. However, the ideal is to reach an agreement through private negotiations, then let the hospital arrange its own publicity to announce the new policy.

Sometimes changes in practices can be introduced by getting the people in authority to agree to a trial period for the new practice. Many groups have found this effective in the area of father-attended births. A committee is set up to draw up an experimental protocol, saying how fathers will be chosen to attend the births, whether they will be required to have preparation, and what evaluation procedures will be followed. Then a trial period is agreed on. Usually by the end of the trial period, the new practice has gained support and acceptance, and the evaluation is positive. In the meantime, those who have been reluctant to accept the new practice have time to observe its effects without feeling that it has been forced on them as a permanent arrangement.

Assuming that you have chosen your issue carefully and done your research thoroughly, the only remaining ingredients for success are time and persistence. You may not reach your goal in time for your currently pregnant members to enjoy the new policies, but the change will certainly occur.

# INDEPENDENCE VERSUS AFFILIATION

Some Cesarean support groups feel strongly that they must be independently organized in order to be most successful. Others feel that organization as a committee of the local childbirth preparation group is more effective, as it lends legitimacy, encourages referrals of Cesarean couples by instructors, and allows the fledgling Cesarean group to take advantage of the experience and material support of the more seasoned childbirth education group. Your group must decide whether independence or affiliation is more suited to its needs. If disagreements do arise between Cesarean support groups and childbirth education groups, they are usually about two issues: The first is that the Cesarean support group may choose tactics that the childbirth group disagrees with, even though the two groups generally agree on goals. The second is that the childbirth education group may wish that the Cesarean group were doing something to stem the tide of the rising Cesarean rate.

With regard to the first, disagreement on tactics, your group can only attempt to negotiate with the larger organization or decide to reorganize independently. No matter what you choose, it is important to decide as quickly and implement your decision as painlessly as possible. Prolonged attempts to resolve these internal problems only serve to divert you from your original goals.

With regard to the second, it may be that your group will choose a project that will affect the local Cesarean rate, such as finding a doctor who will allow a trial of labor following a previous Cesarean. Most support groups consist of people who have already experienced a Cesarean, and their attention and energies are naturally directed to dealing with that fact, rather than with the prevention of future unnecessary Cesareans. The question of which Cesareans are necessary is very complicated, and support groups do not have any obligation to tackle this issue unless they genuinely view it as a priority. By its very existence, a support group reminds the professional community and the public of the tremendous impact that surgical birth has on the family. As members work to educate others, the members also remind them that a Cesarean is not to be chosen lightly.

## NATIONAL AFFILIATION

Three major groups now invite local Cesarean groups to be affiliated with them. (See Appendix I.) Located in Boston, New York City, and Mountain View, California, the groups are similar in their goals, but different in philosophy and tactics. All three make literature available and sponsor informational meetings and conferences. Additional services include leadership training, and a certification program for teachers of Cesarean childbirth preparation classes. Local groups can receive mailings without affiliating formally. Individual memberships are also available, and usually entitle the member to receive the group's newsletter. In most cases, these groups will help you get in touch with someone else in your area, or at least in your state, who is concerned about Cesarean birth. Sometimes regional conferences are sponsored, or at least publicized by these groups. Probably the biggest advantage of contacting such a group is that it provides information and support based on years of experience working to improve Cesarean birth.

> I went to the conference hoping to learn how to get fathers accepted in the delivery room. I did get some ideas, but I also realized how lucky we are around our area. Most women have spinals, and the father and baby join the mother in the recovery room. I heard about places where fathers are just now being allowed to attend *vaginal* births, and everyone who has a Cesarean has a general. It really changed my perspective on things. I also came home full of new energy and enthusiasm.

## PROBLEMS WITHIN THE GROUP

Nobody's perfect, and sooner or later you will have problems among group members. Perhaps there are complaints about the leadership. Sometimes someone joins the group whose personal needs are so great that they interfere with the group achieving its goals; or, since Cesarean birth is associated more highly with problems at birth, there may be one or more members who are contending with a baby who is sick, premature, or who has died. Sometimes groups do not know how to respond to a person with these needs. (See Chapter Twelve, "When Something Goes Wrong.") The variety of internal problems that groups face is endless, and there are certainly no easy solutions. Informal observations tend to show that groups where responsibility is spread among several members come through the inevitable conflicts and discomforts better than groups who depend on a single leader. It also seems that groups that try to solve their problems openly do better than those whose members talk privately, but ignore problems during meetings.

> I finally worked up my courage, when Joanne was talking about her first Cesarean again for the umpteeth time. I said, "Joanne, I have a

problem. I'm feeling very frustrated because I have heard your story so many times, and we have so much business to talk about tonight." She looked kind of upset, and I felt guilty for a minute, but we both lived through it.

## MEASURING YOUR SUCCESS

Since change does occur slowly and requires so much work, it is easy to lose sight of how much you have done. Some changes are so subtle that they can't be measured, such as the difference between the attitudes of people toward your group when it started, versus their increased respect and willingness to listen a year or two later. Other changes come about without anyone being sure why, so you don't know whether to congratulate yourselves or not. For instance, maybe your childbirth educators increased the amount of material they teach about Cesareans even before you had any direct contact with them.

Another, more personal evolution occurs for almost everyone who really gets involved in a support group, and that is a change in your own self-image. You learn that your feelings are not silly and that your problems are shared. You discover that you can understand a great deal of technical material, even without a medical degree. You find an ability to be persistent and assertive that you never knew was there. And you have a greater appreciation for yourself as you experience working and sharing with women who like to work and share with you.

I always used to say that I am not a group person. I guess this was just the first time that I felt so strongly about something that I wanted to get involved. After the next baby comes, I suppose I will move on to other things. But for right now, this is what I want to be doing. Sometimes I watch myself, contacting the papers and generating publicity for the group, talking to people, even being on TV. I never would have predicted this for me, but here I am, and I really like it.

# APPENDIX I

## Nationwide Cesarean Support Groups

Cesarean Birth Association
125 North 12th Street
New Hyde Park, NY. 11040

Cesarean Birth Council
P. O. Box 6081
San Jose, CA. 95150

C/SEC, Inc.
66 Christopher Road
Waltham, MA. 02154

# APPENDIX II

## Other Sources of Support

American Society For Psychoprophylaxis in Obstetrics (ASPO)
1411 K Street N.W.
Washington, DC 20005
One of the two large childbirth education groups. Offers parent and professional memberships. Sponsors teacher certification, newsletters and other literature, regional and national conferences.

Cesarean Connection
P. O. Box 11
Westmont, IL. 60559
Provides a referral service for individuals looking for a Cesarean support group. Their list of groups covers the U.S. as well as some in Canada. Also publishes a monthly newsletter.

Children in Hospitals, Inc.
31 Wilshire Park
Needham, MA. 02192
Support for families of children who need intensive or extended hospital care.

International Childbirth Education Association (ICEA)
P. O. Box 20852
Milwaukee, WI. 53220
One of the two large childbirth education groups. Through education, literature, conferences, etc., supports prepared parenthood. Cosponsors *Birth and the Family Journal* with ASPO.

ICEA Supplies Center
P. O. Box 70258
Seattle, WA. 98107
Stocks a wide variety of literature for parents and childbirth educators on virtually every topic relating to pregnancy, birth, and parenting.

La Leche League International, Inc.
9616 Minneapolis Avenue
Franklin Park, IL. 60131
Disseminates information on breast-feeding. Sponsors local groups and trains group leaders to provide support for the nursing mother. Special help for mothers of premature or sick babies, mothers of twins, and mothers in other unusual situations.

# ANNOTATED BIBLIOGRAPHY

*Birth and the Family Journal.* 110 El Camino Real, Berkeley, CA. A quarterly journal cosponsored by ASPO and ICEA. Current research, reviews of the literature, advertising about recent visual aids, all relating to childbirth and parenting. Three excellent articles from Fall 1977 issue specifically about Cesarean birth are available as bound reprints.

Boston Children's Medical Center. *Pregnancy, Birth and the Newborn Baby.* New York: Delacorte/Seymour Lawrence, 1972.
Very detailed medical information on many issues of concern to parents or parents-to-be. Clear descriptions of common problems, including complications of pregnancy, birth defects, and adjustments to parenthood. Has a bothersome tendency to lapse into referring to pregnant women as "girls." Not available at most bookstores, but worth a trip to the library.

Boston Women's Health Collective. *Our Bodies, Ourselves.* New York: Simon and Schuster, 1973. Paper.
The most thorough book available on women's health care. Contains an excellent section called "The Childbearing Unit." There is essential information on physical, emotional, and sexual aspects of being a woman.

————. *Ourselves and Our Children.* New York: Random House, 1978. Paper.
Why have children, how to raise them, and how to let go. Women and men share the richness of their personal experiences just as members of extended families did years ago. A book to help you know that what has happened to you is probably common, and to help you see what is ahead.

Brazelton, T. Berry. *Infants and Mothers*. New York: Dell, 1969. Paper.
Describes three infants—"average," "active," and "quiet"—in warm terms that encourage parents to accept and appreciate the uniqueness of their baby. Shows how the baby's personality influences parents' behavior.

————. *Toddlers and Parents: A Declaration of Independence*. New York: Dell, 1976. Paper.
Full of the same warmth and respect for parents that is seen in *Infants and Mothers*. Describes common problems: going back to work, sibling rivalry, the toddler's struggle for independence. Discusses how the child learns.

Caplan, Frank (ed.). *The First Twelve Months of Life*. New York: Grosset & Dunlap, 1973.
Good overview of child's development during the first year, complete with photos and growth charts.

C/SEC, Inc. *Frankly Speaking*. 66 Christopher Road, Waltham, MA. 02154. Second Edition. 1978.
So completely expanded and revised that the original isn't recognizable. Contains the best available information and bibliography on vaginal birth after a Cesarean, as well as more general information on Cesarean birth. Highlighted by portions "especially for fathers" throughout the text. C/SEC also has many other publications available.

Dodson, Fitzhugh. *How to Parent*. New York: New American Library, 1970.
Warm and humane approach to the job of parenting. Follows a child through the first five years, pointing out the good and the bad things that are liable to happen along the way.

Donovan, Bonnie. *The Cesarean Birth Experience*. Boston: Beacon Press, 1977. Paper.
The first full-length treatment of Cesarean birth. Lively, sometimes rambling discourse that emphasizes the parents' needs and argues for changes in Cesarean care.

Eiger, M., and Olds, S. *Complete Book of Breast-feeding*. New York: Bantam, 1972.
Talks over basic facts about breast-feeding, as well as mothers who work, relief bottles, and a special chapter for fathers.

Elkins, Valmai Howe. *The Rights of the Pregnant Parent*. New York: Schocken Books; Toronto: Waxwing Productions. Revised Edition, 1980. Paper.
Emphasizes the responsibilities of pregnant parents to become both educated and assertive. Describes how consumers and professionals can become partners. The information is mostly geared toward vaginal delivery. However, the philosophies that Elkins explores are probably even more applicable to the intense and complicated relationship between professionals and the Cesarean family.

Fraiberg, Selma. *The Magic Years*. New York: Charles Scribner's Sons, 1959. Paper.
Offers great insight into the child's perception of her world. Discusses the "mental health" of the developing child. Looks at discipline, punishment, the acquisition of moral values, and many other areas. From a traditional psychoanalytic framework, rises to meet the practical needs of parents in today's world.

Hausknecht, Richard, M.D., and Heilman, Joan Rattner. *Having a Cesarean Baby*. New York: E. P. Dutton, 1978. Paper.
Well-organized and thorough, with a detailed index. Takes a doctor's view, but with an upbeat, proconsumer stance. Some medical errors. Most helpful to those planning a Cesarean.

ICEA. *The Pregnant Patient's Bill of Rights* and *The Pregnant Patient's Responsibilities*. Box 1900, New York, NY. 10001.
Policy statement by one of the two major childbirth education groups about what the pregnant patient may ideally expect, and what she must give in return. Excellent background for parents-to-be who are consciously thinking about and planning for their roles as health care consumers.

Kelley, Marguerite, and Parsons, Elia. *The Mother's Almanac*. New York: Doubleday, 1975. Paper.
From making play dough to dealing with clutter, all done with wry humor. Wonderful understanding of the differences in ability and comprehension among children from two to six. An essential survival manual.

Klaus, Marshall H., and Kennel, John H. *Maternal-Infant Bonding*. Saint Louis: The C. V. Mosby Company, 1976. Paper.
Describes the original research that led to the current intense interest in bonding. Excellent chapters for professionals and for all who wish

to support parents of premature children, children with birth defects, and grieving parents. Critical comments from many other professionals incorporated into the text.

La Leche League International, Inc. "Breastfeeding After a Cesarean." 9616 Minneapolis Avenue, Franklin Park, IL. 60131. Revised, 1978. Or contact your local La Leche League chapter.
Practical hints and birth reports from Cesarean mothers.

Lansky, Vicki. *Feed Me, I'm Yours*. New York: Bantam, 1974. Paper.
Healthful, uncomplicated recipes for preschool children from six months on. With the help of this book, you may even find your children eating vegetables.

Levine, James. *Who Will Raise the Children: New Options for Fathers (and Mothers)*. New York: Bantam, 1977.
Examines fathers who have elected to spend at least half their time as "housepersons."

Lowe, John A., M.D., et al. "Cesarean Sections in U. S. PAS Hospitals," *PAS Reporter*, Vol. 14, Dec. 1976.
Commission on Professional and Hospital Activities, 1968. Green Road, Ann Arbor, MI. 48105.
The best compilation of data regarding Cesarean deliveries that is currently available. Statistics relating Cesarean rate to hospital size, region of the United States, etc. Examines rates of complications to mother. Charts and graphs on every page.

McBride, Angela Barron. *The Growth and Development of Mothers*. New York: Harper & Row, 1973.
Stresses the importance of the mother growing along with her child. Discusses how a mother can help her child develop more fully by being aware of the important issues in the mother's own life.

MacFarlane, Aidan. *The Psychology of Childbirth*. Cambridge, MA.: Harvard University Press, 1977. Paper.
A complete review of the research on mothers and babies. Properly read, it will stimulate your imagination but impress you with how little we know with any certainty. Lovely description of the abilities of the newborn. No material specific to Cesarean birth.

Montreal Health Press. *Birth Control Handbook* (11th ed.). P. O. Box 1000, Station G, Montreal, Quebec H2W 2N1, Canada.
Simple language but complete information on birth control.

Noble, Elizabeth. *Essential Exercises for the Childbearing Year*. Boston: Houghton Mifflin, 1976. Paper.
Exercises specifically designed for Cesarean women during the immediate postpartum time. Good program for the entire year—pregnancy and recovery. Clear illustrations.

Prendergast, Linda C., and Rosno, Suzanne. *Cesarean Beginnings: A Handbook for Parents and Professionals*. Beginnings Publications, 1548 Johnson Avenue, Saratoga, CA. 95070.
The best of the half-dozen or so booklets now available. Complete, includes professional opinions in support of father-attended Cesareans, class outline for Cesarean birth classes, and extensive reading list.

Rozdilsky, Mary Lou, and Banet, Barbara. *What Now? A Handbook for New Parents*. New York: Charles Scribner's Sons, 1975.
Excellent book for all new parents. One chapter devoted specifically to Cesarean birth. Practical and humorous advice on how the novice can survive and even enjoy parenting.

Schiff, Harriet. *The Bereaved Parent*. New York: Viking/Penguin, 1978. Paper.
The only full-length book for parents who have lost a child. Relates experiences ranging from the loss of an infant to parents whose child has died after reaching adulthood. Looks closely at the mourning process and the effects of grief on marriage, friendships, and other children. The author speaks from personal experience. Lacks specific treatment of the unique problems faced by the parents of a child who dies at birth or soon after.

Schultz, Terri. *Women Can Wait: The Pleasures of Motherhood After Thirty*. New York: Doubleday, 1979.
Describes the joys and trials of waiting until you have accomplished more of your own growth before you undertake to oversee the growth of a child.

Spock, Benjamin. *Baby and Child Care*. New York: Pocket Books, 1968. Paper.
The basic book of parenting, like an encyclopedia in its scope. You may not always agree, but you will find that Dr. Spock has something to say on virtually every topic. Very sympathetic toward parents. Extremely helpful for those moments when you don't know if you should call the doctor or hope the problem will disappear on its own.

# Index

Abdominal tightening exercise, 131
Abruptio placenta, 33–34
Acceptance, as response to
  Cesarean delivery and problems,
  191–92, 206–7, 229–31
Acupuncture, 65
Afterpains, 240
Age, maternal, choice of delivery
  and, 37–38
American Academy of Pediatrics,
  114
American Society for
  Psychoprophylaxis in Obstetrics
  (ASPO), 281
Amniocentesis, 33, 37, 39, 55–59;
  *ill.*, 58; problems of and
  alternatives to, 57–59
Amniotic fluid (amniotic sac), 101,
  102, 106; amniocentesis and,
  55–59; rupture of the membranes
  and (*see* Rupture of the
  membranes)
Anemia, 41
Anesthesia, 65–78 (*see also*
  Anesthesiologist); choice and
  kinds of, 65–70 (*see also* specific
  kinds); father-attended birth and,
  259–60; pre-op and delivery
  preparation, 82, 96, 97
  professional preferences and
  policies and, 66–68; recovery
  from, 125–27
Anesthesiologist, 18, 66, 67–68, 70,
  272 (*see also* Anesthesia); and
  delivery, 94, 95, 96, 97; and
  father-attended birth, 252, 253
Anger, as response to Cesarean
  delivery and problems, 172,
  183–84, 206, 219, 225–26
Antacids, use of, 88
Antibiotics, use of, 88–89. *See also*
  Penicillin
Apgar scores, 106–7; chart, 107
Aspiration, general anesthesia and
  problem of, 71, 88; antacids and,
  88
"Assessment of Continuous Fetal
  Heart Monitoring in Labor, An,"
  (Kelso, et al.), 49n

Atropine, use of, 88

*Baby and Child Care* (Spock), 287
Baby, birth of, 101–2. *See also*
  Delivery
Baby carriers, use of, 161; Huggle
  Bunny, 161
Bassinet, portable, 161
Bathing, post-delivery, 138–39, 157;
  showers, 138–39; tub, 157
"Belly binders," 134–35
*Bereaved Parent, The* (Schiff), 287
Bicornuate (two-chambered) uterus,
  25
"Bikini." *See* Transverse skin
  incision
*Birth and the Family Journal*, 283
Birth control, 8, 158, 176–77, 286.
  *See also* Sterilization; Tubal
  ligation
*Birth Control Handbook*, 286
Birth defects, 203, 204, 207–20;
  causes, 219; and infant death
  (*see* Infant death); statistics, 204
Birth experience, postpartum
  understanding of, 143–46
Bladder, recovery and, 128
Blood (blood problems, blood
  supply): placenta previa and,
  31–33; pressure (*see* Blood
  pressure); Rh disease, 40–41;
  tests (*see* Blood tests);
  transfusions, 41
Blood-gas determinations, fetal,
  51–52
Blood pressure, checking, 84, 96;
  high (*see* Hypertension); low
  (*see* Hypotension)
Blood tests (blood samples): estriol
  levels, 61–62; fetal monitoring
  and, 50, 51–52; of newborn
  infants, 108–9; pre-op, 83
"Blues, the," after-delivery, 141
Body temperature, newborn infants
  and, 111
Bonding. *See* Parent-infant bonding
Books (annotated bibliography,
  283–87)